LANGUAGE ACQUISITION IN THE BLIND CHILD

Language Acquisition in the Blind Child

NORMAL AND DEFICIENT

Edited by
ANNE E. MILLS

CROOM HELM
London & Canberra

COLLEGE-HILL PRESS
San Diego

©1983 Anne E. Mills
Croom Helm Ltd, Provident House, Burrell Row,
Beckenham, Kent BR3 1AT

British Library Cataloguing in Publication Data

Language acquisition in the blind child.
    1. Children, Blind   2. Perception in
    children   3. Communication Psychological
    aspects.
    I. Mills, Anne E.
    362.7'95   HV1598
    ISBN 0−7099−1768−6

COLLEGE−HILL PRESS, INC.
4580−E Alvarado Canyon Road
San Diego, California 92120

Library of Congress Cataloging in Publication Data
Main entry under title:

Language acquisition in the blind child.

    Papers originally presented at an international
symposium, held Sept. 1981 in Tübingen, Germany.
    1. Children, Blind−−Congresses. 2. Children, Blind−−
Education−−Congresses. 3. Children−−Language−−Congresses.
4. Verbal learning−−Congesses. 5. Language disorders
in children−−Congresses. I. Mills, Anne E.
HV1596.2.L36   1983   401'.9   83−1917
ISBN 0−933014−89−9

Printed and bound in Great Britain

CONTENTS

Tables and Figures
Preface
Notes on Contributors

1. EDNA ADELSON
    Precursors of Early Language Development
    in Children Blind from Birth............   1-12

2. HENNING WODE
    Precursors and the Study of the Impaired
    Language Learner.......................   13-17

3. WALTER ELSTNER
    Abnormalities in the Verbal Communica-
    tion of Visually-impaired Children......   18-41

4. CHRIS SCHANER-WOLLES
    Speech Therapy for the Blind...........   42-45

5. ANNE E. MILLS
    Acquisition of Speech Sounds in the
    Visually-handicapped Child.............   46-56

6. BARBARA DODD
    The Visual and Auditory Modalities in
    Phonological Acquisition...............   57-61

7. BARBARA LANDAU
    Blind Children's Language is Not
    "Meaningless".........................   62-76

8. PAUL WERTH
    Meaning in Language Acquisition........   77-88

9. RANDA MULFORD
    Referential Development in Blind
    Children................................ 89-107

10. HARRY McGURK
    Effectance Motivation and the Develop-
    ment of Communicative Competence in
    Blind and Sighted Children............ 108-113

11. CHARITY ROWLAND
    Patterns of Interaction between Three
    Blind Infants and Their Mothers........ 114-132

12. TON VAN DER GEEST
    Cognition, Interaction, and Develop-
    ment, with Special Reference to the
    Education of the Handicapped Child..... 133-141

13. CATHY URWIN
    Dialogue and Cognitive Functioning in
    the Early Language Development of Three
    Blind Children......................... 142-161

14. MICHAEL GARMAN
    The Investigation of Vision in Language
    Development............................ 162-166

15. SUSANNE MILLAR
    Language and Active Touch: Some
    Aspects of Reading and Writing by Blind
    Children............................... 167-186

16. RICHARD F. CROMER
    The Implication of Research Findings on
    Blind Children for Semantic Theories
    and for Intervention Programmes........ 187-196

References.................................... 197-214

Author Index................................. 215-220

Subject Index................................ 221-235

TABLES AND FIGURES

Tables

3.1 Percentage of Visually-handicapped
    Children with Language Disorders ...   25
3.2 Percentage of Visually-handicapped
    School-beginners with Language Dis-
    orders   25
3.3 Distribution across Age Groups of Lan-
    guage Disordered Visually-handi-
    capped Children at the Time of Dia-
    gnosis from Kindergartens I and II .   29
3.4 Categorization of Children in Kinder-
    gartens I and II according to Social
    Class   35
5.1 The Visual Groups of Consonants Tested
    by Mills and Thiem (1980)   47
5.2 Elicited Imitations of Syllables from
    One Blind Child (Hanna) and One
    Sighted Child (Joanna)   51
5.3 Substitutions in Spontaneous Utter-
    ances from One Blind Child (Hanna)
    and Two Sighted Children (Joanna and
    Amahl) which involved Consonants
    from Visual Group 1 (/b/, /p/, /m/)   53
5.4 Substitutions in Spontaneous Utter-
    ances from One Blind Child (Hanna)
    and Two Sighted Children (Joanna and
    Amahl) which Involved Consonants
    from Visual Group 2 (/f/, /v/)   54
6.1 Percentage Inattention to In- and Out-
    of-synchrony Presentation   58
6.2 Comparison of Blind and Sighted Chil-
    dren's Phonology   60
8.1 The Semantic Distinctions between
    Verbs of Perception   83
11.1 Subject Profile   117

11.2 List of Coded Behaviours 121
11.3 Comparison of Pairs on Occurrence of
      Selected Behaviours: Proportion of
      Intervals Containing Each Behaviour 122
11.4 Examples of Spontaneous Manual
      Gestures 123
11.5 Magnitude and Z_{sums} of Crosslagged
      Functions 126
11.6 Pre- and Post-project Scores on Com-
      municative Skills Interview 129-30

Figures

3.1 Frequency of Language Disorders among
     Children in Pre-school Institutions
     for the Blind and Partially-sighted
     Compared with Sighted Children   27
3.2 Frequency of Language Disorders among
     Visually-handicapped Pre-school
     Children according to Sex and
     Kindergarten   28
3.3 Comparative Frequency of Language
     Disorders in Totally Blind and Par-
     tially-sighted Pre-school Children .   30
3.4 Proportional Distribution of Language
     Disorders in Blind and Partially-
     sighted Compared with Sighted Pre-
     school Children   32
3.5 Comparison of Phonological/Phonetic
     and Morphological/Syntactic Disor-
     ders in Totally Blind and Partially-
     sighted Boys and Girls   33
3.6 Comparison of Phonological/Phonetic
     and Morphological/Syntactic Disor-
     ders amongst Boys and Girls in
     Kindergartens I and II   34
3.7 Causes of Difficulties in Verbal Com-
     munication in Visually-handicapped
     Pre-school Children   38
7.1 Early Vocabulary of Two Blind Subjects
     Compared to Sighted Children   65
7.2 Early Sample of Semantic-syntactic
     Relations Expressed by Two Blind
     Subjects Compared to Sighted Chil-
     dren   67
7.3 Later Sample of Semantic-syntactic Re-
     lations Expressed by Two Blind Sub-
     jects Compared to Sighted Children .   68

15.1 Mean Latencies for Correct Responses by Blind and Sighted Children to Appropriate and Inappropriate Adjective-Noun Word-Pairs Taken from Four Modalities of Perception 169

15.2 Simplified General Visual Reading Model 171

15.3 The Proportions of Errors for Helen and Blind Subjects A, B and C on Successive Letter Matching with Verbal, Spatial and Texture Interference 177

15.4 The Proportion of Errors and Latencies for Correct Responses in Retarded and Non-retarded Braille Readers in Successive Matching of Braille letters according to Format 180

15.5 Simplified Tactual Braille Reading Model 183

PREFACE

Anne E. Mills

The papers published in this volume were first presented at an international symposium[1] "The Development of Language and Communication in the Blind
Child" held in September, 1981 in Tübingen, Germany.
The topic may seem a specialized one, yet it is of
importance within several disciplines. Contributions to the symposium came from the fields of education and medicine as well as psychology and linguistics. Such meetings are also rare and those who
do research in this area are separated both by distance and by the academic frontiers of the disciplines involved. In bringing these researchers together the aim of the symposium was not only to pool
results but to encourage inter-disciplinary cooperation, thus giving the work in this area a broader
and sounder theoretical basis.
    Some of the chapters are predominantly a report
of results from work from blind children. These are
of interest in themselves since so little is known
about the early learning of blind children. Other
chapters contain a more general discussion of the
critical issues raised by such research and emphasize the relevance of findings from the blind to
theories of language acquisition.
    A general issue which recurs throughout this
volume is the question why we should study the language of blind children at all. It is not enough to
state merely that we want to know what happens in
the language acquisition of a handicapped group; it
is important to formulate a clear motivation.
    Taking a theoretical perspective, we can use
evidence from the blind child to evaluate the role
of vision in the language acquisition of sighted
children. This is the perspective predominant in
the chapters by Mills and Mulford. Under the assumption that all other things are equal (which they

are usually not, see the chapter by Elstner), the blind child faces the task of acquiring language with one missing source of information, the information gained through vision. In theories of language acquisition in sighted children, the role of vision is in fact more often implicit than explicit. The evidence from blind children is therefore of general interest since it helps define the role of vision in language acquisition, and therefore provides a more precise account of the language development process. This perspective, as McGurk (see Chapter 10) rightly points out, does not, however, help the blind child any further.

Vision may have different roles in development. In the case of blind children following the same developmental path as sighted children, any explanation based on the use of vision must be rejected. If the blind child follows the same developmental path but is slower in his development, vision must be accorded a stimulating factor. If the blind child arrives at the same point but follows a different developmental path from the sighted child, any explanation of acquisition must put vision in relation to the alternative sources of information the blind child uses. As Urwin (see Chapter 13) and Millar (see Chapter 15) discuss, the loss of vision may not necessarily be a handicap.

Obviously, in order to evaluate the language acquisition of the blind child in terms of such aspects as structural differences, functional differences and differences in input, we must be able to put our findings in relation to development in the sighted child. Despite the vast amount of research carried out in the last decade in this area, we often do not have enough information to make a clear comparison. This lack of information makes it very difficult to interpret the findings from blind children, as is evident for example in the chapter by Rowland on interaction. This is especially critical when trying to evaluate whether any differences which may be found between blind and sighted children constitute a risk for the language development and general development of the blind child. It is this information which the therapist needs to have in order to come to a founded decision on intervention. Will differences in input, for example, have a clear effect on the language produced by the child and how important is any resulting difference in the child's language for his continuing development? It may be of no relevance at all; it may be crucial.

The therapist needs to know how to assess any

such deviations in order to determine the necessity of intervention. This is important in all assessments of intervention, as Schaner-Wolles discusses (see Chapter 4), not only with the blind child. The therapist also needs to know what the role of vision is in language acquisition, so that, where deviations attributable to lack of sight occur, alternative compensatory means of presenting the necessary information can be found.

As mentioned above, it is rarely the case that all other things are equal, that is that blindness is the only handicap. According to the evidence presented in the chapters of this volume, it would seem that blindness alone is not sufficient to produce deviant language acquisition. Where blindness comes together with other handicaps of whatever kind, the chances of language disorders are increased. It is therefore necessary to know how to compensate for the lack of vision in order to reduce the effects of other handicaps.

As stated earlier, the contributors to this volume come from a variety of disciplines and represent different standpoints, that of the practitioner concerned with intervention and that of the theorist concerned with explaining language acquisition in general terms. This volume is also intended to be of interest both to those readers working with blind children and to those who have a general interest in language acquisition.

Finally I should like to thank Laura Lane for her help in translating some of the contributions and Gabriele Weiss and Ruth McEwan for their help in preparing the manuscript for publication.

NOTES

1. The symposium was supported by a grant from the Deutsche Forschungsgemeinschaft and the State of Baden-Württemberg.

NOTES ON CONTRIBUTORS

Edna Adelson is Assistant Research Scientist in the Child Language Project at the University of Michigan, Medical Center, Ann Arbor, Michigan, USA.

Richard F. Cromer is a Research Psychologist at the MRC Cognitive Development Unit, London, England.

Barbara Dodd is Lecturer at the School of Education, University of Newcastle-upon-Tyne, England.

Walter Elstner is Speech Therapist at the School for the Blind, Vienna, Austria, and Chairman of the School Committee of the International Association of Logopedics and Phoniatrics.

Michael Garman is Lecturer at the Department of Linguistic Science, University of Reading, England.

Barbara Landau is a Sloan Postdoctoral Fellow in the Department of Psychology, University of Pennsylvania, Philadelphia, USA.

Harry McGurk is Senior Lecturer at the Department of Psychology, University of Surrey, Guildford, England.

Susanna Millar is Research Officer in the Department of Experimental Psychology, University of Oxford, England.

Anne Mills is Lecturer in the Department of English, University of Tübingen, West Germany.

Randa Mulford is Postdoctoral Fellow at the Institute of Child Development at the University of Minnesota, Minneapolis, USA.

Charity Rowland is Director of the Family Focus Research Project, The Morrison Center, Portland, Oregon, USA.

Chris Schaner-Wolles is Lecturer in the Department of Linguistics, University of Vienna, Austria.

Cathy Urwin has a research position in the Child Care and Development Group, University of Cambridge, England.

Ton van der Geest is Professor in the Department of Dutch Language and Literature, Groningen University, The Netherlands.

Paul Werth is Chargé de cours at the Free University of Brussels, Belgium.

Henning Wode is Professor in the Department of English, University of Kiel, West Germany.

Chapter 1.

PRECURSORS OF EARLY LANGUAGE DEVELOPMENT IN CHILDREN
BLIND FROM BIRTH

Edna Adelson

THE ROLE OF VISION IN EARLY DEVELOPMENT

A ten-year study of normal delays and detours in the
development of infants blind from birth[1] led us to
insights about the role of vision in the processes
and organization of early development. We also
gained an appreciation of the unique adaptive problems faced by the blind infants, their families, and
the research clinician.

The central findings of the research are summed
up by Selma Fraiberg in Insights From the Blind
(1977, pp. 282-3):

> We were able to facilitate the blind infant's
> development in every sphere of development, but
> the impediment of blindness could be discerned
> at every point in development at which repre-
> sentational intelligence would lead the sighted
> child into the organization of an object world.
> We could facilitate the affective ties to human
> partners, but the constitution of those part-
> ners as objects was delayed by comparison with
> sighted child norms. We could facilitate the
> coordination of hand and ear, but this coordi-
> nation was still dependent upon the blind
> child's ability to attribute substantiality to
> persons and things when only one of their at-
> tributes, sound, was given. We facilitated
> locomotion but we could still discern the
> impediment to locomotion, the absence of the
> distant lure usually provided by vision, the
> reach for 'something out there'. We saw that
> blindness was not a major impediment to the
> acquisition of language in the first two years
> of life when we were able to maximize the
> experience of the blind child and his language

1

environment. But the impediment of blindness
revealed itself in an impoverished dialogue and
in the protracted delay in the constitution of
a stable concept of *I*.

In our view, language acquisition has its
beginnings in the sensorimotor period, for blind as
well as sighted infants. For the young blind child,
who must apprehend the world without vision, there
is an especially close link between communication
and the quality of available experience in prehension and locomotion, and between the extreme
difficulties in the establishment of object permanence, and the vicissitudes of human attachment.
Our study began with the assumption that strong
human attachments would create the essential context
for reciprocity and communication between infant and
parent. Then, as daily events created a world that
was interesting, predictable and enjoyable, infant
and parent would have things to talk about, to tell
each other. Our task as researchers and clinicians
was to decode non-verbal and pre-verbal sets of
communications so that the child was not held back
from progress toward representational intelligence,
language, and abstract and imaginative thought.

THE CASE-STUDY OF KAREN

The problems of Karen and her family present a com-
pelling example of aborted communication, a failed
dialogue. The family's difficulties also highlight
the problems usually posed by blindness and point to
the role of vision in linking partners to one another, in building pathways to a world of objects,
words and ideas, in integrating varieties of
experience.

Factors Determining Developmental Delay
Karen is blind. When I first saw her at eleven
months, her parents described her as being "no
trouble at all" - and so she was, since she slept
20 hours a day and did little but suck her pacifier
when awake. She seldom laughed or cried or vocalized. She did not like to be held and was unhappy
except lying in her baby bed or sitting in her
bouncing seat where no toys could be kept within
reach. The back of her head was bald. Her hands
looked peculiar and useless. Most of the time they
were up near her shoulders, bent back at the wrists,

2

half closed. Occasionally when she was upright, she
swept at the space behind her head in a strange,
apparently purposeless way. She presented a fright-
ening example of a failure to progress after months
of unintentional maternal and sensory deprivation.

Mr. and Mrs. Cook are a stable working class
couple who were then in their early twenties. They
told me the story of her birth and blindness.
Karen, their first child, was three months premature, weighing only two pounds three ounces, and it
was two months before she could come home from the
hospital. Her worried parents tried to hold her
then, but she was stiff. She seemed to reject their
attention and she did not look at their faces. She
was not the way they expected a baby to be, and they
could not understand what was wrong. Soon Mrs. Cook
became pregnant again. After a while they wondered
if Karen could see and they took her to a doctor who
insisted that nothing was the matter. Not until
Karen was four months old was the blindness
officially confirmed and diagnosed as retrolental
fibroplasia, a condition which can be caused in
premature babies by the supplemental oxygen used in
the incubator. She was totally blind.

When Karen was just eight and a half months
old, her sister Patty was born, also premature, but
not quite as small. Patty spent one month in
hospital. Mr. and Mrs. Cook were faced again with
fears about a tiny infant and possible blindness,
and had nowhere to turn for help.

In spite of their anxiety and fear, they did
what they thought was right for both children. They
bathed and fed them and kept them quiet. They described infancy as a dull time when babies only eat
and sleep, and that was what the girls did. As
Karen's first birthday drew near, they waited
patiently for her to walk and talk, but were
beginning to doubt that she would. A pediatric
ophthalmologist who examined Karen then referred the
family to the Child Development Project.

On visits to the home to observe and assess
Karen and to offer information and support to Mrs.
Cook, I also saw Patty. Watching her, I came to
understand what Karen's first year may have been
like. Patty was not blind, but her days were
monotonous and lacking in stimulation. Within the
walls of her cot or tilted back in her infant seat,
she had nothing to look at, nothing to play with.
Her bottle was propped up beside her. She had too
much sleep, too little handling. She rarely made
any vocal sounds. I made suggestions and brought

3

her toys but they were not used. She began to show
similarities to the institutionalized babies described by Provence and Lipton (1962). At seven
months an attractive toy was dangled before her.
She looked at it silently. She moved towards it
eagerly with her eyes, her mouth, her head, but her
hands remained out at her sides; she did not even
begin to reach for it.

Patty was deprived and delayed in many ways, as
we suspected Karen had been. Nevertheless, her
future was not in jeopardy to the same extent because she was not blind. She could see her parents
and something of the world around her. She was
cuddly and comprehensible to her family, and when
she grew too big and active to be contained in an
infant seat any longer, she began to reach and move
toward what she saw, and came alive - a little late,
but definitely on her way.

For Karen such an easy change was impossible.
For a blind child the world will not suddenly reveal
itself after eleven impoverished months. Instead
the natural increase in motor energy is more likely
to lead to repetitive dead-end behaviours which are
not definitely due to blindness, since they also
occur in disturbed sighted children. Such behaviours establish themselves as the understimulated
blind child attempts to adapt to restricted and
fragmented experience (see Smith, Chethik and
Adelson, 1969).

We already had a fair grasp of early ego development in the blind. Details of our research and
educational programmes are reported elsewhere
(Fraiberg, 1977). Briefly, we have found that the
milestones of human attachment should be as they are
for any child: smiling, preference for the mother,
reaction to a stranger, all being shown at the usual
times. Sleeping and eating patterns and early
speech patterns should also be no different. Crawling and walking are usually delayed in the blind
child, but good control of the body in other ways
should not be late. Since touch and hearing do not
automatically compensate for the missing sense of
sight, special care must be taken to ensure from the
start that the hands come together at midline, that
the fingers become adept and alert, and that sounds
come to have meaning. An important finding of our
research is that 'reach on sound' (see Fraiberg,
1977, pp. 162-8), which is as important to the blind
child as 'reach on sight' is to the sighted child,
may not occur until ten or eleven months of age,
that is five to six months later than 'reach on

sight'. Until it does occur, there will be no
attempt to seek something out of reach, no crawling
or mobility.

Our central concerns are to establish and support the emotional tie between parent and child, and
to build in essential learning experiences of hand
and ear during the prolonged period of immobility
when the blind infant cannot seek them himself, when
his special needs may be misunderstood or under-
estimated.

We had been able to do this for blind infants
whom we saw very early in the first year. Would it
be possible to help Karen? In this case report I
will touch on each of the developmental areas that
prompted our research interest and clinical concern.

Development of Non-Verbal Dialogue

Karen's appearance at eleven months and her parents'
reports about her infancy sounded too much like
other descriptions and histories in the literature
on the disturbed child, for example from Provence
and Lipton (1962). Although no developmental scales
have been standardized for infants totally blind
from birth, we knew from our own research sample and
from the study by Norris, Spaulding and Brodie
(1957) that Karen was functioning at a seriously
retarded level. However, there were several indications that change might still be possible. Firstly,
her mother and father cared very much for her and
were seeking help. Secondly, there was no evidence
from recent medical examinations to indicate other
handicaps or brain damage. More important was what
we saw in Karen herself. Karen had reacted strongly
to her mother's absence at the time of Patty's
birth; she had slept even more, eaten less, and her
vocalizations had almost stopped. To us this meant
she responded to and missed her mother and she was
attached in some way. She did smile when spoken to.
Her muscle tone was good as she sat in her bouncing
seat. Even her awkward hands offered hopeful cues;
they did come together to hold her bottle. When I
left my hand beside hers, I could feel her fingers
move very slightly on mine in tentative exploration.
She did not reject the outside world but she had not
yet discovered it.

We had to find some way to bring mother and
baby together, to let them begin to share small
spontaneous moments with pleasure. Nevertheless I
always had to respect the family's own style. The
home visits, which lasted an hour, were once a week

for a while and then twice monthly. The sessions were filmed monthly. The notes taken during the visits and films were summarized and reviewed by the project staff.

Firstly, we noted that Karen would let me hold her for play, but that she was seldom held by her mother. We thought the regular bottle feedings might be a route to bring about change. If Mrs. Cook could hold Karen, then they would have many times together each day. Mrs. Cook listened politely while I described what it meant to a child to be held close, listening to her mother's voice as she enjoyed her bottle, to touch and to be touched, to hear and to be heard. But she continued her routine of propping Karen's bottle beside her and leaving her alone to drink it. When I pressed Mrs. Cook to feed Karen on her lap while I was there, she did so, but mother and child were clumsy, stiff with apprehension. Mrs. Cook looked stoney and cold; Karen looked blank, empty. This was not going to work at all, so I had to rethink my strategy.

Somehow I had to find a bridge between mother and child without usurping Mrs. Cook's central role. On each visit I spent a few minutes sitting on the floor to play with Karen on my lap. I introduced her to the toys I had brought, while making my own unobtrusive assessments. Karen enjoyed these play sessions. Maybe this would be a way Mrs. Cook could more easily hold and enjoy her child, but she was making no moves in this direction. She remained depressed and doubtful. One morning, as Karen played with a bell on my lap, she made some small sound which I firmly said meant that she wanted her mother. Somehow I stood up with Karen and the bell and the toy box and deposited them all on Mrs. Cook's lap. Through it all Karen continued her fascinated exploration of the bell. Mrs. Cook, in her intuitive effort to balance everything, enclosed Karen in her arms and soon was drawn into the play herself. She pulled on the bell gently and held Karen fast; their heads touched and they both smiled. They were comfortable with each other and together they went on to explore the rest of the toys. It was a start. Playing with toys, with its possibilities of active exchange, and demonstrations of intelligence did the trick. A dialogue of play was possible. A dialogue with words was yet to come.

Development of Verbal Dialogue

Mrs. Cook was shy and found conversation a strain. She seldom spoke to Karen to tell her what was happening. It was difficult to convince her that Karen paid attention to her mother's words, that Karen could use language to make sense of an invisible world. The natural course of events provided a clear demonstration. The family dog was scolded all day long. The sudden sharp commands made me flinch every time. One day, just as Karen learned to sit by herself on the floor, the dog wandered by and Mrs. Cook shouted angrily *Get out of here!*. Karen froze, trembled, and began to cry. I comforted her and she resumed playing. Later, a fierce warning was again shouted at the dog, but this time the dog's name had preceded the shout. Karen quieted for a moment, but she did not seem afraid and she did not cry.

There was small hope of getting Mrs. Cook to stop scolding the dog. Perhaps this regular event could prove useful. I commented on the two episodes and asked Mrs. Cook to let me know how Karen reacted at other times. Did she notice a difference when the dog's name was used? Intrigued by Karen's potential cleverness, Mrs. Cook tested it completely before the next visit. She reported with great satisfaction that Karen had never cried when the dog was scolded by name. Her parents were impressed and life became a little more predictable for Karen. Through this occurrence, Karen also became more predictable to her parents. Mrs. Cook said Karen thought about a lot of things and understood more than you might guess.

Conceptual and Motor Development

After four weekly visits, several changes indicated to us that Karen's daily routine was improving and that her parents were more assured of her adequacy. When Mrs. Cook recognized Karen's boredom, she no longer treated it as fatigue and did not hurry her to bed. As a result Karen's sleep decreased dramatically. She took only two naps and her bald spot faded. Her hands had not yet relaxed but she rolled about and could get onto her hands and knees. She sat comfortably on her mother's lap and could also sit unsupported on the floor. This was considerable progress, but her parents could not understand why she did not try to crawl or walk right away.

Like most people, Karen's parents could not understand the unique conceptual problems faced by a

7

blind child. It takes more effort, more time to
organize inner and outer experience without vision
to aid memory and to confirm and reconfirm what is
perceived. For example, how did Karen make sense of
the space around her and her place in that space?
An interesting clue lay in the odd sweeping gesture
Karen made behind her head when she was standing up.
For several weeks, it remained a puzzle. Then, one
day, after Karen had lost her uneasiness about playing on the floor, she was lying on her back shaking
a rattling cube when it fell from one hand landing
beside her ear. She moved her arm repeatedly back
and forth between her shoulder and head trying to
grasp the cube which she could feel with her fingertips. Karen, with many months of experience on her
back, was conducting a perfectly good search based
on past successes with fallen bottles and pacifiers.
    I did not appreciate what all this meant until
later during the same visit. After Karen had played
with a musical rattle while supine on the floor, I
took it from her and sounded it beside her. Lured
by the musical note, she rolled over onto her stomach. I shook the rattle in front of her. Karen
accurately located the rattle by the sound, stretch-
ed her arm straight toward it, touched it with her
fingertips but could not quite grasp it. This reaction confirmed that her physiological maturation
had advanced, that refined hearing was now available
to her which she could use for reality testing, communication, and self/object differentiation. Her
subsequent curious behaviour however revealed her
mental dilemma. Instead of reaching again to the
spot where she had just felt the rattle, Karen bent
her arm and brought it back to sweep the space between shoulder and head. It was another attempt at
a search and it was quite useless under the circumstances. Yet she repeated the movements, even after
the rattle was sounded again and she had reached
forward once more to touch it. Her behaviour
appeared senseless, irrational to us, yet it made
sense to Karen. In Karen's limited world, there was
only one place to find things. She knew that in her
bed fallen things always landed on the mattress towards her back. Although the floor was now beneath
her stomach, she continued to direct her search towards her back. She could unite sound and touch and
infer the rattle's existence outside herself, yet
she could not appreciate the new relationship between her body, the floor, and the toy. Words alone
could not help her with this puzzle.
    Karen needed time to learn the new possibili-

ties of her own body. She needed to learn that, if
she reached out through the darkness and the silence, there was much to be found at her fingertips.
She needed to enjoy play that would give her reliable and accurate mental images of the outer world.
We lent the family a playpen and for the next month
Karen used this enclosed space to discover what she
needed to know about herself and about inanimate objects. With the playpen I left some toys: one from
a toy store, one I had made, one an ordinary kitchen
item. Mrs. Cook caught on. By the next visit she
had bought a better toy, invented a more interesting
gadget, and found many kitchen things that Karen
liked. Mrs. Cook was also sure Karen preferred
those her mother chose for her. Led on by her interest in all these new playthings, Karen thoroughly
explored the possibilities within the playpen. She
learned that what was out of reach remained near by
on the mat or higher up on the rail. It now made
sense to search persistently and in different ways
for what she wanted and, as she searched, she moved
ever more efficiently, first on her stomach, then on
hands and knees. While she played, she babbled. She
was able to pull herself up to a standing position,
and she would always initiate these activities herself.

For the next half year, Karen made progress in
many areas. Gross motor changes were rapid and much
valued by the family. At 13 months, Karen crawled
across the living room. One month later, she knew
the entire house. Her mother said, "I never know
where she is now." Soon she was climbing into
everything. At 17 months, she took her first steps,
and by 18 months she preferred walking to crawling.
She was upright and active.

Changes in Karen's hands came more slowly. For
almost half a year her grasp remained clumsy and im-
mature, a very visible sign of progress still to be
made. Mrs. Cook was encouraged to engage Karen's
hands at midline with toys or hand play, but these
suggestions met with little or no reaction from the
mother. They may have called for more physical
intimacy than Mrs. Cook could tolerate. She liked
to keep things picked up, so that no toys were left
lying about. When Karen left the playpen to roam
the house, she found few playthings. Nevertheless,
I could see that Karen's hands were gradually becoming more adept at seeking and learning.

Another reassuring change occurred. As soon as
Karen became active and mobile, the sweeping gesture
near her head disappeared. Gradually she brought

her hands down from shoulder level, and they became
more open. But when there was momentary confusion
around her, as, for example, when a stranger
approached or when her mother scolded her sharply,
her hands went briefly back to the old posture and
became a signal to us that she was uncertain or
afraid. If Karen's development had not been altered, it is likely these behaviours would have per-
sisted in their inutile forms. Seen several years
in the future, they would have been difficult to understand, and even more difficult to change. They
would have been tagged as undesirable habits or
blindisms.

Development of an Emotional Tie and Language
In this same half year, other very important advances were occurring which alternatively pleased
and confused the Cooks or which revealed continuing
conflict. Earlier Karen's parents had felt rebuffed
and hurt by her stiffness and unresponsiveness. Now
Karen could make her feelings quite clear. She made
it obvious that she was not about to share attention
or playthings with her sister Patty. When Patty was
out of reach in the playpen, Karen shouted and
fought to get toys away from her. And just as
clearly Karen showed she could not do without her
mother whom she would follow or seek over any distance and around any obstacles throughout the house.
    Karen's move toward her mother was wholehearted
and her love and longing were unmistakable to me.
Her mother's reaction to this was cautious. Sometimes I spoke for Karen, expressing what I thought
she felt when she looked happy or seemed sad, always
calling her mother's attention to these reactions.
I repeatedly pointed out how Karen smiled at her
mother's voice and quieted to mine. I also spoke to
Karen, telling her how delighted I was when something I did pleased her, how discouraging it was
when I did not know the right thing to do. Karen
listened and babbled. Mrs. Cook did not participate
in these 'conversations', but gradually she could
bring Karen closer to her. When Karen was teething
or had a cold, her mother could take her on her lap
to comfort her without words and Karen snuggled
close. Mrs. Cook began to ask Karen what she wanted
or what she meant. Karen picked up the questioning
tone and would say *whatsit?* or *whosit?*, when she
touched or heard things.
    At 14 months Karen tried to stay near her
mother, crawling after her, playing beside her,

clinging to her. She then began to show normal
separation anxiety and could not be left with rela-
tives or friends when her mother shopped. The Cooks
felt Karen was becoming spoiled and needed stricter
treatment and more separations. I explained that
Karen was making up for what she had missed; when
she could hold her parents more permanently in her
mind, she would move away at her own pace. With
this explanation, Mr. and Mrs. Cook were able to
give Karen the close contact she needed through this
period. By 16 months, she was more tolerant of
strangers and had less need to know constantly where
her mother was. At 17 months her mother was set
free as Karen took off on her own, eager to explore
new situations. She was independent and confident.
She was at last walking on her own. To her parents
this meant she was all right. A month later, for
the first time, I heard Mrs. Cook identify herself
as *Mama* to her child.

It was in the delayed use of this word *Mama*,
and in the reluctant acceptance of Karen's attempts
at speech that Mrs. Cook's continuing hurt, doubt,
and anger towards Karen showed itself. Karen's
language was the last accomplishment to meet with
her mother's recognition and approval. From what
Mrs. Cook reported, Karen's vocalizations had dete-
riorated in the months before I first saw her. She
had once cried loudly for long spells. Unable to
understand or to comfort her, her parents had left
her alone in her cot until she quieted. She had
once babbled and even shouted the baby sounds she
knew, but when I first saw her she neither laughed
nor cried. Only a few whispers were the sum of her
earlier babbling behaviour.

Slowly, as Karen became more responsive and
comprehensible, her mother began to speak to her.
She spoke loudly, almost as if she thought a blind
child could not hear well, and the loud voice seemed
to express a natural anger. It was interesting to
note that, when Karen resumed babbling at 13 months,
it was with the same angry intensity one heard in
her mother's voice. Karen had two words at 1;1.23.
She could ask for things at 1;2.7 (tickle game). At
14 months Karen would obey the inhibiting command *no
no*. At 15 months she 'talked' all the time in
babbled sentences which had little detectable meaning but contained fine conversational inflections.
She acquired two new words for family members, *Da-da*
and *Sissy*, but no word yet for mother. Karen's
father always found some meaning in what she said
and judged her as talking quite well. Her mother,

not yet hearing her own name from her child, judged her as hardly talking at all.

I could hear Karen's new words and questions clearly. However, most of her attempts to speak were ignored by her mother. Mrs. Cook's response was always *What did you say? I can't understand you.* Suggestions were made of other ways in which one might respond to Karen, but at that point Mrs. Cook was not able to support her child's language development. When Karen was two years old, she began to say *Mama.* From that point on, Mrs. Cook could hear and understand the other things Karen said. Finally, when Karen was two and a half, her mother began to talk comfortably to her, picking up her phrases or questions and giving answers that led Karen into more speech. From then on Karen's speech improved rapidly. She never merely echoed what was said to her. She had two-word sentences at 2;2.13. She quickly mastered the use of *I* and *you* by 2;11.0. In fact, her use of language became quite impressive compared to the other blind children we were following (see Fraiberg, 1977).

SUMMARY

By the age of 18 months Karen's condition was much improved and by 24 months we were even more assured of Karen's adequacy. She was able to enjoy new experiences and integrate the new into a growing repertoire of adaptive behaviours. She and her mother had many dependable ways to communicate. She could walk. She could talk. Corcrete experiences could be described in words. Her parents took hope and were proud of her. Dialogue that suited this particular family was possible once we could clarify the distortion and delay in each sphere of non-verbal sensorimotor development. Karen was preparing the foundations for stable memories and for abstract and imaginative thought. Without any vision, all this was difficult but it was possible.

NOTES

1. "The Early Ego Development of Children Blind from Birth" was a study carried out at the Child Development Project at the University of Michigan and was mainly supported by the National Institute of Child Health and Development during 1966-71 (Grant No. HDO1-444). Selma Fraiberg was Director and Principal Investigator.

Chapter 2.

PRECURSORS AND THE STUDY OF THE IMPAIRED LANGUAGE LEARNER

Henning Wode

Why should we study the acquisition of language by impaired subjects, for example by blind children? From her case study of Karen, Adelson (Chapter 1.) makes clear the importance of intervention and therapy in promoting the development of the blind child. I wish here, however, to consider some of the theoretical issues which the study of blind children's development raises, particularly in relation to language. Three important issues emerge in my opinion from Adelson's paper. The first issue is a methodological one, that is the suitability of studying a handicapped group, in this case the blind, as a research paradigm to gain insights into the process of acquisition in unimpaired learners. The second issue is the problem of integrating the findings from such a research paradigm in the general development of the field. The third issue revolves around the concept of 'precursor' with respect to language learning. The first and second issue I will discuss together since they are interrelated. The third issue will be discussed separately.

THE IMPAIRED LANGUAGE LEARNER

Most modern studies of language learning have two deficiencies: a. they do not in general refer to the impaired learner, whatever the nature of the impairment, and b. only children learning their first language are studied. As the following brief summary will show, however, these deficiencies reflect the history and development of the field. At the beginning of research on language acquisition around the turn of the century, the focus was on monolingual children, although there were some

attempts to include bilingual children, for example
by Ronjat (1913), Pavlovitch (1920), or Leopold
(1939-1949). Unimpaired children were investigated
primarily, although there has been the occasional
exception, for example Jakobson's (1941) study of
aphasic patients in relation to the development of
phonology. However, even after the revival of
interest in child language research during the
1960's due to the advent of transformational grammar, the focus remained fixed on first language (L_1)
acquisition by unimpaired learners.

During the late 1960's and early 1970's a major
breakthrough occurred, in that other acquisitional
types besides L_1 were studied. Research on second
language (L_2) acquisition in a naturalistic setting
was one of the first new types to be established as
a field worthy of investigation. Since then, it has
become increasingly clear that the fields of investigation could no longer be restricted to either L_1
or L_2 acquisition or even to the study of acquisition in small children. Language acquisition needs
to be studied in its entirety, that is in all types
of learners, of all ages and in all learning situations, for example, learning a language in a classroom, forgetting a language and relearning it etc.
The insights which have already been gained from
this reorientation of the field have required drastic revisions of many views popular both among lay-
men and researchers. It is now questioned, for
example, whether adults learn a language in a totally different way from children. Language learning
in the classroom is not to be clearly separated from
learning outside the classroom. The similarities
that exist in all types of language learning situation call for an integrated view (for details and
references see Wode, 1981).

Moreover, I think that the most important insight derived from this reorientation is that
language learning seems to require specific types of
cognitive ability or abilities which cannot be
equated with general intelligence, the rise of logical thinking, or the various stages of intellectual
development as laid out, for example, in Piagetian
psychology. This is where it becomes methodologi-
cally almost imperative to broaden the range of
investigational options to include language learning
by the impaired.

Learning a language means essentially processing speech input in order to extract from it the
rules of the target language. Unimpaired learners
are likely to make use of the whole range of

cognitive and sensory mechanisms at their disposal.
It is therefore difficult to identify or observe
with precision the exact contribution of each of the
individual components of this processing system as
long as they are activated together. If, however,
some components cannot be activated, as is the case
with impaired learners, then the effect(s) of the
components can be studied directly by identifying
the differences when compared to unimpaired learners. It should be obvious that this provides an excellent opportunity to determine with a greater
degree of sophistication what may be due to perceptual processing via the senses as opposed to some
more deep-seated cognitive component. Moreover, it
is clear that to achieve this the kind of impairment
should be identified as precisely as possible, as
argued by Schaner-Wolles (Chapter 4). Little will
be achieved by broad groupings, such as impaired
versus unimpaired learners. For example, there are
studies on deviant phonology where various etiologies are lumped together (e.g. Ingram, 1976). It is
necessary to conduct studies relative to specific
etiologies.

Apart from such general considerations, it
seems to me that the study of the blind learner may
prove to be a landmark in the development of the
field. For example, the preliminary report from the
project conducted by Anne Mills at Tübingen on phonological acquisition by blind children (Mills,
Chapter 5) convincingly shows that some of these
phonological peculiarities relate to specific visual
(dis)abilities and not, as one may have been in-
clined to suspect, to some more deep-seated cognitive abilities that might govern language learning.
Similarly, the work by Barbara Landau (Chapter 7),
Randa Mulford (Chapter 9) and Catherine Urwin
(Chapter 13) makes one wonder why people might have
ever entertained the idea that the acquisition of
certain discourse skills, of reference, and of the
meaning of certain lexical items should not heavily
depend on the ability to see.

In short, then, it seems that the study of impaired learners is likely to enrich and refine im-
mensely our understandings of how human beings learn
languages. I hope that such studies will, eventually, also be conducted on blind adolescents and adult
L_2 learners.

PRECURSORS

The concept of 'precursor', which Edna Adelson discussed, is, in my opinion, an extremely important notion and raises issues which I would like to expand on here. As I see it, there are three possible interpretations of the notion, namely the metamorphic interpretation, the place-holder interpretation and the catalyst interpretation.

According to the metamorphic interpretation, the precursor stands in relation to the subsequent phenomenon as a seed to the adult plant, that is the precursor, as a phenomenon, develops into the subsequent phenomenon through a process of metamorphosis.

According to the place-holder interpretation, a phenomenon A prepares the ground for phenomenon B but there is no metamorphosis of A. To illustrate this in language, a child may use at some stage a non-target-like construction, such as *no* in negation in English in, for example, *I no want envelope* 'I don't want an envelope'. Such a construction is then later replaced by a more target-like structure, in this example when *don't, didn't* start to be used. *Don't* and *didn't* do not however appear to be metamorphized forms of *no* (see Wode, 1977).

According to the catalyst interpretation, the precursor triggers a reaction without being affected itself at all. In language acquisition a phenomenon B will not occur unless phenomenon A has first occurred. For example, learners of German tend not to use the phoneme /ö/, as in *schön* 'beautiful' before /i/, as in *Dieb* 'thief'.

The notion of precursor is extremely important with respect to the cognition issue, that is when thinking about the relationship between cognition and language learning. This issue tends to be discussed primarily in terms of Piagetian theory of cognitive development. Piaget, as is well known, never made language acquisition his object of study. He was interested in how children learn a language as an indication of general intellectual development. It is becoming increasingly clear of late that the kind of cognitive development envisaged in Piagetian theory of child development does not explain those aspects of language acquisition that relate to the structure or properties of the linguistic devices, such as word order, inflectional marking, embedding etc. (see Wode, 1981 for a detailed discussion). Therefore, either the place-holder interpretation or the catalyst interpretation

would seem to be most plausible in describing the relationship between general cognition and language. The metamorphic interpretation would seem highly im- plausible since the formal properties of the lin- guistic devices would have to be accounted for as growing out of general cognitive operations. The precursors of the linguistic devices, within this interpretation, would have to be formal operations which would be quite different from Piagetian formal operations and which I would want to call linguo- cognitive abilities. The kind of interpretation given to the notion of precursors needs to be care- fully considered when studying language learning, particularly when dealing with the impaired learner.

To summarize then, it would seem that the study of impaired learners promises to lead us to a much clearer understanding of the nature of those capaci- ties that underlie the functioning of man's senses and abilities as they relate to the complex phenom- ena of learning natural languages. Moreover, it seems that research on impaired learners promises to make our understanding much more precise with re- spect to the contribution of the individual senses. And it may also be the case that our traditional thinking about what may have been a precursor needs to be reversed. It is quite possible, for example, that the ability to see promotes certain develop- ments in language learning, but, on the other hand, that the absence of sight leads to the extension or more speedy development of other language capaci- ties.

Chapter 3.

ABNORMALITIES IN THE VERBAL COMMUNICATION OF
VISUALLY-IMPAIRED CHILDREN

Walter Elstner

DEVELOPMENT OF LANGUAGE IN THE VISUALLY-HANDICAPPED:
AN OVERVIEW

According to prevailing views, the basic principles
of general human development also apply to children
with limited sensory perception or children who have
lost the use cf a particular sense, as in the case
of blindness. Of course, such handicaps create particular conditions for development. The important
factors here are the point at which the handicap began and the seriousness of the handicap. When
serious visual disorders begin at an early age, for
example, the entire physical and mental development
is altered (Solnzewa, 1975, p. 304). Language development and language abnormalities can only be
understood within the framework of development as a
whole. Such a description of the development of the
blind child has been provided by Solnzewa (1975,
1977, 1980, 1981), among others. The studies of
Fraiberg (1974) and Wills (1979), referred to below,
are also informative.

The Development of Communication

Children come into contact with their social environment long before they master the sound system of
their language. Pre-linguistic means of communication developed at this time, which later become elements of communicative behaviour together with the
sound system, function via the various senses and
the motor system. At this stage, two aspects of the
reciprocal emotional exchange become evident: that
of 'being addressed' and that of 'addressing'. It
is critical for the blind infant that he lacks the

18

visual triggers for making mutual contact and can
only develop compensatory behavioural patterns gradually.

The sighted infant has already developed a
large repertoire of visually-determined behavioural
patterns by the age of six months. He uses the
"smile language" (Fraiberg, 1974, p. 222) and the
differentiated "eye language" (Fraiberg, 1974;
Argyle, 1980). The blind child, on the other hand,
has no way of watching his mother's facial expressions or of observing the joint and simultaneous
nature of visual and auditory events. Consequently,
he misses valuable stimuli for speaking; he remains
poor at expressing himself and loses many communicative opportunities.

Let us also consider the perspective of the
sighted people in the blind baby's environment.
They unconsciously expect the culturally predeter-
mined reactions and behaviour patterns of sighted
babies, which would act as the trigger for their
affectionate responses towards the child (Fraiberg,
1974, p. 221). They therefore misinterpret the
blind baby's expressionless face as reflecting rejection or lack of interest. As Wills (1979, p. 89)
formulates it, the child and the world around him
communicate "on different wavelengths". Fraiberg
(1974, p. 226) drew attention to the hands of the
blind child, however, which do serve as an adequate
means of expression and are indicative of an active
mind.

One of the early means an infant has of establishing contact is to produce sounds. The blind
infant, however, seems to take less advantage of
this than the sighted infant, since auditory stimuli
cannot be connected with visual stimuli to form perceptual complexes on a higher level. This is the
reason, according to Fraiberg (1974, pp. 226-9),
that blind children rarely initiate any "vocal
dialogues" themselves, even under favourable environmental conditions. The blind infant learns at an
early age "to distinguish voices, but they come from
the unknown and return to the unknown"[1], (Solnzewa,
1980, p. 36). Thus, blind infants remain dependent
on the initiatives of the people around them. Perhaps this is the root of later isolation (Rogow,
1972, p. 36).

The Acquisition of Concepts and Meanings

Semzowa (1961) has demonstrated that, among young
blind school children, one cannot expect an increased sensitization of the remaining senses.
Rather one finds, if anything, a certain decrease
in comparison with the sensory perception of comparable sighted children (Lux, 1933; Elstner, 1955).
The auditory threshold for blind children, for example, hardly differs from that of sighted children
(Semzowa, 1961, p. 338). Studies of conceptual
development in young school children are informative
in this connection (Semzowa, 1962, pp. 30-7). These
results show that blind children have most difficulty in distinguishing concepts which refer to activities or spatial relationships. The fact that they
also have difficulty in the representation of concrete objects was established by Solnzewa (1975,
p. 306). In this study, young pre-school-age blind
children could only identify 27.7 per cent of the
objects presented to them, whereas a comparable
group of sighted children achieved 100 per cent with
the same objects. Without sight, the "great organ-
izer of perception" (Wills, 1979, p. 91), the
remaining senses are much less capable of making
sense of the environment. The child who cannot see
finds it difficult to abstract the information which
is essential, for example, for the recognition of
people, animals and objects, for understanding the
course of events and their relationship to one another, and for orienting himself. He can rely only
on the use of the senses of hearing, touch, and
smell. These difficulties lead to a deficit in concrete representations, and as a consequence to a
lack of interest in an external world whose signals
cannot be united into meaningful entities. For this
reason, help on the part of caretakers, teachers,
etc. at an early stage, especially in the motor
development of the blind child, is of extreme importance (see Solnzewa, 1977, p. 107, among others).

With the beginning of language, the blind child
gains a tool for the expansion of his conceptual
world. The time of greatest development for the
blind child who is not multiply-handicapped is
between 1;6 and 5;0 (Solnzewa, 1977, p. 107). His
first verbal utterances are above all a means of
communication with the people in his environment
(Solnzewa, 1981, p. 233). Many blind children show
an increased ability in imitating speech sounds, and
later words and word combinations, especially if
they are of the "auditory type" as defined by

Mansfeld (1952, p. 48). This ability is also positively reinforced by an affectionate response from
the child's caretaker. The use of language for
purely communicative purposes, however, is an obstacle to the acquisition of concrete reference in language. Since the blind child is severely limited in
terms of the physical area in which he lives, the
danger exists of perception in the auditory mode remaining distinct from perception in the other modes.
This may be the explanation for the finding that
blind children remain at the stage of echolalia for
a prolonged period (Wills, 1979, p. 116; Rogow,
1972, p. 37), and tend to so-called 'verbalism'. At
a later stage, if the conceptual content of utterances is incomplete, tasks are solved on a purely
verbal basis (Solnzewa, 1977, p. 108).

The Development of Morphology and Syntax

In the previous section, it was argued that the main
difficulty for blind children of normal intelligence
lies in comprehending the concrete nature of verbal
expressions and differentiating between concepts;
they appear, however, to acquire formal structures
with relative ease. Solnzewa (1980, p. 38) reports
that blind children imitate sounds from their surroundings, such as animal voices and the noise of
engines etc., later than sighted children, but
speech sounds earlier. This willingness to imitate
also lasts longer and, as mentioned above, can lead
to echolalia at a later stage. As discussed earlier, the blind child's early language is primarily
communicative in nature. It is also characterized
by the playful manipulation of sounds, phrases and
compounds. Wills (1979, p. 112 ff) illustrates this
playfulness with many examples from her observations
of the linguistic development of two blind children.
For these children, speech sounds acquire a life of
their own (Wills, p. 112). The speech of blind
children is much more freewheeling and independent,
and not so restricted by the constraints of meaning
as the speech of sighted children (Wills, 1979,
p. 86).

The sound of some patterns and combinations in
language greatly fascinates certain blind children.
Their production of such patterns then triggers off
the production of new similar-sounding combinations
through a process of association. Wills (1979) describes many examples of this behaviour. I, myself,
taped a ten-year-old girl many years ago, who played

with such sound patterns and put them into song form. This playing with sounds also occurs in the context of speech therapy. The therapy consists of practicing particular combinations of consonants in nonsense syllables with different vowels. This phonetic training, which usually inspires great merriment among the children, gradually earns the title of 'fun exercises'; it picks up on the children's own enjoyment of sound games. Often the children vary the basic material with similar-sounding examples from the sound patterns they are familiar with from the spoken language. It is conceivable that children with an auditory orientation first acquire grammatical structures and syntactic sequences as sound patterns and only gradually assign content to them.

The level of concrete, direct language that the blind child needs in order to cope with life around him, lags somewhat behind his control of formal structures acquired through sound patterns. Wills (1979, p. 113) describes one of the children she observed who, in spite of a high syntactic level in his "freewheeling" language, could not express his real needs verbally, and was largely dependent on his mother's help. The other child observed by Wills could produce longer sentences. However, he was not able to construct these himself, but produced exact repetitions of what he had heard. He had learned these utterances as whole sentences from their sound structure.

Phonological Development

It has been reported that a sighted infant can already imitate mouth and tongue movements at the age of two months (Trevarthen, 1974). That the sighted child babbles over an extended period is common knowledge. The blind child, on the other hand, babbles much less (Fraiberg, 1974, p. 229). The absence of visual stimuli in the pre-verbal stage seems to be responsible not only for the lack of babbling, but also for particular phonological characteristics and the large number of articulatory mistakes among young blind children.

Typical examples of these mistakes, observed by many authors, are the tentativeness or lack of precision in the articulation of particular phonemes, although this inaccuracy rarely impairs communication. Instances from German are the bilabial formation of /v/ and the interchanging of /m/ and /n/ (eg. *Mikolaus* instead of *Nikolaus* 'Father Christmas')

or of /st/ and /sp/, in either initial or final position (Lux, 1933; Elstner, 1955 and 1966; Häusler,
1968). Mistakes in English include the substitution
of /l/ or /r/ for /w/, /ʃ/ for /s/, /ð/ and /θ/ for
/f/, and /n/ for /m/ (Fladeland, 1930; Wills, 1979).
Kostjutschek (quoted in Solnzewa, 1975, p. 307) made
similar observations about Russian. Göllesz (1971)
reports deviant lip articulation among Hungarian
blind children. In a study of 14 blind pupils in
the Budapest School for the Blind, he established
that blind children show more lateralization and
less movement of the lower lip than sighted pupils.

Mills and Thiem (1980) recently investigated
the interaction of visual and auditory information
in the perception of speech sounds. They define
four visual categories of German consonants which
play an important part in determining perception
under experimental conditions and which can function
as aids in discrimination under normal conditions.
The fact that these discriminatory aids are not
available is a possible explanation for the high
number of phonological abnormalities among visually-
impaired children. This is discussed in more detail
in Mills' paper (Chapter 5).

Rogow (1973, p. 107 ff) points out that blind
children often have less sensorimotor experience in
the area of the mouth. They generally 'explore'
various objects with their lips and tongues much
less than sighted children. This is significant not
only for lexical and semantic but also for phonological development. One must also consider the
finding, which is confirmed by our own observations,
that blind children are often fed solid food at a
much later point than sighted children. The con-
sumption of solid food requires differentiated chew-
ing and swallowing movements which function also as
the precursors of articulatory movements.

In the preceding remarks, I have shown that
even a blind child who is not multiply-handicapped
is exposed to certain dangers in his development. A
healthy environment can avert these dangers to a
large extent and can effectively help compensate for
the adverse effects of blindness. These effects are
critical, however, for multiply-handicapped blind
children or for children who grow up in an unfavourable milieu. This explains the fact that in many of
the studies which deal with the verbal abilities of
blind children, such a large percentage of speech
abnormalities is observed.

LANGUAGE ABNORMALITIES AMONG BLIND AND PARTIALLY-SIGHTED CHILDREN IN SCHOOLS FOR THE BLIND

Incidence of Language Abnormalities

Before starting the discussion proper, I wish to mention briefly the problem of defining any abnormality in language. Baumgarten (1979, p. 73)[2] gives the following definition:

> Linguistic behaviour is labelled abnormal by the individual himself or by the people around him, when it deviates from the various language norms defined by social groups or authorities. Language may be abnormal on phonological-articulatory, morpho-syntactic, or lexical-semantic levels. Depending on the nature of the abnormality, the individual will suffer a handicap not only in his ability to act on the world but also in the areas of cognition, emotion, psycho-motor ability and social learning.

This is, in my opinion, the most complete definition as yet produced and covers the kind of abnormalities found in blind children very well. By using the term 'language abnormality' one avoids classifying the behaviour prematurely as a specific disorder. The term 'disorder' is moreover used in widely differing ways by different authors, so that a comparison of different findings is problematic.

Some of the authors who study the mental development of blind children also report the presence of, what they call, speech disorders. According to most studies, more than 40 per cent of the children have speech abnormalities, when different age groups are studied.

The following table shows the percentage of children with speech disorders reported in various studies. These statistics, however, are not strictly comparable. Stinchfield (quoted in Maxfield, 1928, p. 71) investigated the entire population of blind children including pre-school children and the educationally-subnormal in Philadelphia and Watertown, the largest institutions for the blind in the United States. Miner (1963) studied seven- to sixteen-year-old blind and partially-sighted[3] pupils at schools in Michigan and Illinois. Häusler (1968) examined school-age pupils at eight German schools for the blind, including both blind and partially-sighted children. He excluded, however, children in vocational schools, the educationally-subnormal and

pre-school children. Elstner (1971), like Stinchfield, studied the whole population of pupils at the
Vienna school for the blind. This institution is
only for the totally blind, since there is a special
school in Vienna for the partially-sighted.

Table 3.1: Percentage of Visually-handicapped Children with
Language Disorders

Author	Period of Data Collection	Language Disordered (%)	Population (n)
Stinchfield	1923, 1925	49	404
Miner	1961-2	33.8	293
Häusler	1967	45.25	411
Elstner	1969-70	44.27	131

Source: Stinchfield (1928), Miner (1963), Häusler (1968),
Elstner (1970)

In 1971, the author also carried out a more
limited study of the blind children just starting
school, and compared his results with those of
German and Soviet investigations. The results are
presented in Table 3.2. As would be predicted, the
figures relating to language-disordered children
were somewhat higher than they were for the population as a whole.

Table 3.2: Percentage of Visually-handicapped School
Beginners with Language Disorders

Author	Period of Data Collection	School Beginners – Language Disordered (%)	Population (n)
Elstner	1969-70	57	102
Semzowa & Solnzewa	1962-3	40	62
Häusler	1967	62	53

Source: Elstner (1970), Semzowa and Solnzewa (1966), Häusler
(1968).

The highest incidence of language disorders was found among pre-school children, especially pre-school multiply-handicapped children. I will discuss these groups in the following sections.

In contrast to the studies which report a higher occurrence of language abnormalities among visually-handicapped children than among sighted children, the investigations of Fraiberg (1968, 1974) and Wills (1979) show almost no speech disorders among congenitally blind children, but just a somewhat retarded speech development. According to Brieland (1950), the difference between the speech of blind and sighted children is also small.

These apparent contradictions can be explained when one considers the fact that the results here are taken from observations of completely different groups. Reports of non-deviant language development come from congenitally blind children or children blind from an early age with no further disorders, and who have developed in an optimal milieu. Experience at the school for the blind has taught us, however, that such children are the exception. The majority of children in schools for the blind have not had such favourable social conditions, and a large number of them have further primary or "consecutive disabilities" (see Bracken, 1969[4]). Not one of the 93 children in the author's study had had the advantages of the same favourable conditions as the children observed by Fraiberg or Wills.

The diversity of individual circumstances makes it impossible to draw statistically valid conclusions. No two children are exactly the same with regard to those variables which are significant for mental and physical development, and therefore also for linguistic development. The following list summarizes the variables already mentioned earlier:

- degree of visual faculty (total or partial blindness)
- time of onset of visual impairment (congenital blindness, blind since early childhood etc.)
- cause of the visual impairment
- age of child (infant, pre-school child, school-age child)
- additional disorders (deafness, mental or physical handicap, learning disorder, minimal cerebral palsy, emotional and/or behavioural disorders)
- social factors (social class, neglect/overprotection, hospitalism, suitable training - especially at an early age).

The incidence of a multiple-handicap is far higher than blindness alone and is strongly associated with a language disorder. In the past few years, questions about the education and development of multiply-handicapped children have been debated with increasing frequency. In particular, the pronounced increase of minimal cerebral palsy and the ensuing handicaps is a topic of current discussion (Benesch, 1974).

Classification and Relative Frequency of Language Abnormalities

My own work at the Vienna Institute for the Blind will be described here in more detail in relation to the kinds of abnormality that occur, their relative frequency and the factors associated with an abnormality in language development. Only those abnormalities are counted here which required speech therapy. The study is limited to children at pre-school age attending the two kindergartens[5] (KG I, KG II) of the Institute between 1970 and 1981. The populations are described in Figures 3.1 and 3.2. Diagnosis was made on school entry.

Figure 3.1: Frequency of Language Disorders among Children in Pre-school Institutions for the Blind and Partially-sighted Compared with Sighted Children

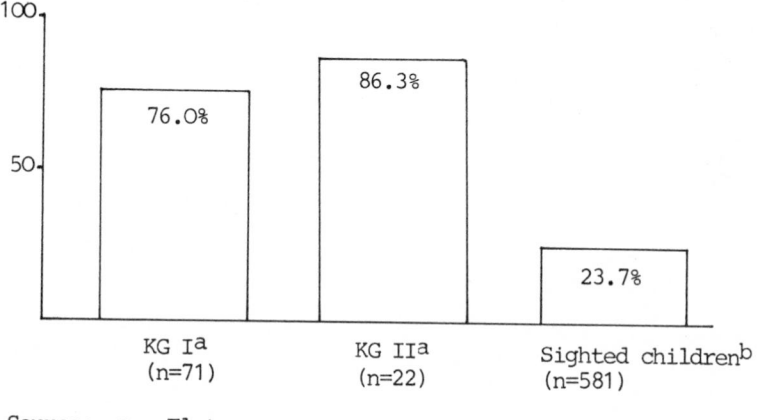

KG I[a]
(n=71)

KG II[a]
(n=22)

Sighted children[b]
(n=581)

Source: a. Elstner
Source: b. Hess (1955)

Figure 3.2: Frequency of Language Disorders among Visually-handicapped Pre-School Children According to Sex and Kindergarten.

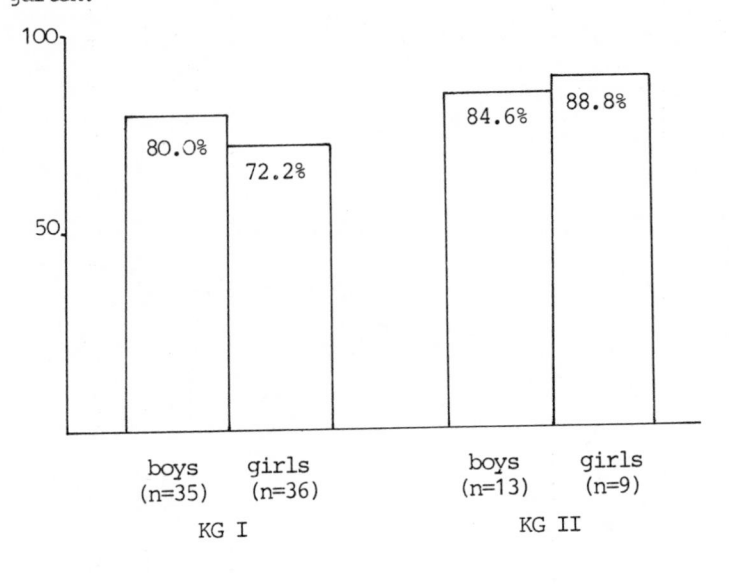

    Comparison in the number of disorders (Figure 3.1) is made with a group of sighted children from kindergartens in Lucerne, Switzerland, investigated by Hess (1959, p. 201). Table 3.3 gives the age structure of the children studied.
    It is striking that pre-school children in the Vienna Institute for the Blind (KG I and KG II) have a higher frequency of language disorders than the comparable group of sighted children, and that the children in Kindergarten II (KG II) have more language disorders than the children in Kindergarten I (KG I). These two findings were to be expected, since, firstly, earlier studies have found that blind and visually-handicapped children have had more language disorders than sighted children. Secondly, language disorders are more frequent in younger children and children with additional handicaps (Elstner, 1955, 1966, 1971; Häusler, 1968).

Table 3.3: Distribution across Age Groups of Language Disordered Visually-handicapped Children at the Time of Diagnosis from KG I and KG II

Age[a] (years)	Totally Blind		Partially Sighted		Total
	Boys	Girls	Boys	Girls	
3	1	2	1	1	5
4	4 (1)[b]	7 (1)	0	2	13 (2)
5	8 (2)	9 (3)	3 (1)	2 (1)	22 (7)
6	8 (3)	4 (2)	3 (1)	4	19 (6)
7	3	1 (3)	3	1 (1)	8 (4)
8	0	0	2 (1)	1	3 (1)
9 and older	2	0	1	0	3
Total	26 (6)	23	13 (3)	11 (2)	73 (20)
Mean Age	5.7 (5.3)	4.8 (7.3)	6.4 (6.3)	5.4 (6.0)	5.6 (6.2)

Note: a. It will be noticed that some of the children are older than school age (6 years in Austria). In certain circumstances it is possible for a child to remain in a kindergarten, for example when there is difficulty in making a clear diagnosis of the child relevant to determining his future education.

Note: b. The figures given in brackets refer to the visually-handicapped children with no language disorder, for the purpose of comparison.

Classification according to sex (see Figure 3.2) reveals an almost equal frequency of speech disorders among boys and girls. According to the data from sighted children, one would have expected a higher incidence (almost double) in boys than in girls.

Surprisingly, a further classification of the results according to degree of visual faculty showed a higher occurrence of language abnormalities among the children with partial vision than among those who were completely blind (see Figure 3.3). Earlier studies (Häusler, 1968; Elstner, 1971) have found the reverse relationship, that is that totally blind children show a greater incidence of language disorders than the partially-sighted. Among the partially-sighted children in this study, there are a large number of multiply-handicapped and educationally-subnormal, so it can be argued that this sample is not representative of the whole population of partially-sighted pupils at schools for the blind.

Figure 3.3: Comparative Frequency of Language Disorders in Totally Blind and Partially-sighted Pre-school Children.

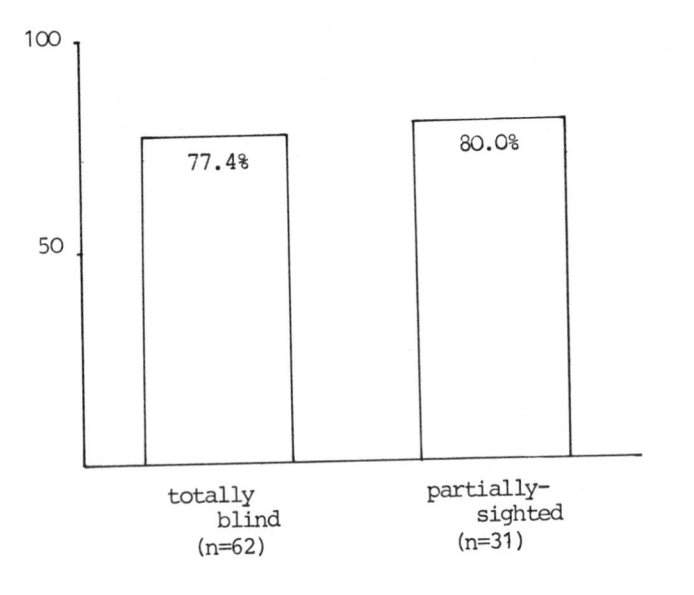

Following is a survey of the proportions of different types of language disorders within the total number of language abnormalities (= 100%) which were found among completely blind and partially-sighted pre-school children (see Figure 3.4). Again, the statistics from Hess about sighted kindergarten pupils are given for comparison. Disturbances in the flow of speech (stuttering and cluttering), which have not previously been mentioned, are also included. Neither these nor the abnormalities listed under 'other disorders' (nasality and vocal impairments, among others) are considered to be important in view of disorders in language development in general, so they may be disregarded here.

It appears that the morpho-syntactic and lexical-semantic abnormalities, when compared to the phonological-phonetic abnormalities, account for a greater proportion of disorders among blind and partially-sighted children of pre-school age than among sighted kindergarten pupils. Phonological-phonetic abnormalities constitute approximately half of all disorders among blind and partially-sighted children, whereas they make up three quarters of sighted children's disorders. The difference between the visually-handicapped and sighted children in terms of disorders in morpho-syntactic development is even more pronounced; approximately one third of all disorders are of this type among visually-handicapped children, compared with only four per cent among sighted children. This leads one to the conclusion that visually-handicapped children have particular problems with the structural and semantic aspects of language in comparison with sighted children.

As is to be expected, many of the visually-handicapped children had multiple language disorders. Almost all children with disorders in morpho-syntactic development also had problems with articulation. It is of course not possible to determine if phonological abnormalities occur among the children with 'almost no speech'. They are 'potential' stammerers, however, since their poor ability to differentiate phonemes only improves gradually, even when favourable results are obtained in therapy.

Figure 3.4: Proportional Distribution of Language Disorders in Blind and Partially-sighted Children Compared with Sighted Pre-school Children

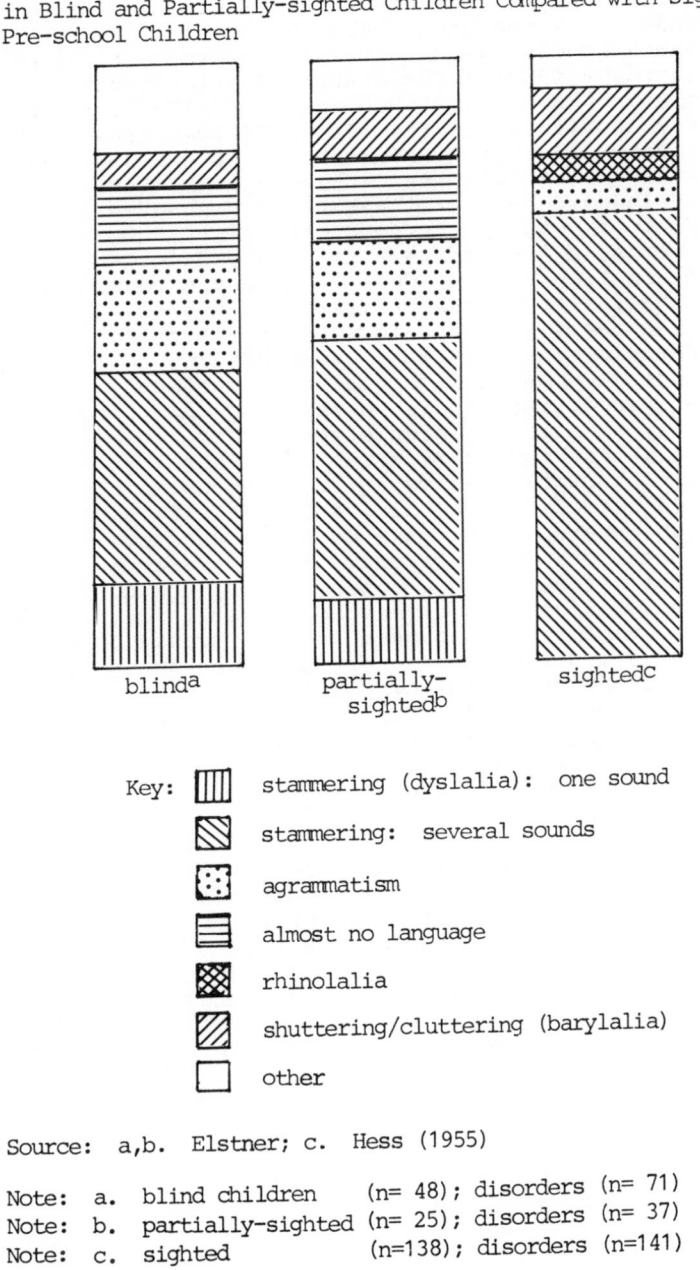

blind[a] partially-sighted[b] sighted[c]

Key:
- stammering (dyslalia): one sound
- stammering: several sounds
- agrammatism
- almost no language
- rhinolalia
- shuttering/cluttering (barylalia)
- other

Source: a,b. Elstner; c. Hess (1955)

Note: a. blind children (n= 48); disorders (n= 71)
Note: b. partially-sighted (n= 25); disorders (n= 37)
Note: c. sighted (n=138); disorders (n=141)

32

In Figure 3.5, the two language abnormalities, 'stammering: single sound' and 'stammering: several sounds', are combined under the heading phonological-phonetic disorders, and are compared with the two disorders in morpho-syntactic development, 'agrammatism' and 'almost no speech'. The figures from the two kindergartens (I and II) were combined; the children were grouped according to sex and visual faculty (totally blind - partially-sighted). As was mentioned above, it was to be expected that children with the greatest loss of vision would have the most disorders in every aspect of language tested. The only result of this comparison which agreed with predictions was the relationship between completely blind and partially-sighted children in terms of morpho-syntactic abnormalities: completely blind children had proportionally more morpho-syntactic abnormalities than children with partial vision. All other comparisons did not match predictions.

Figure 3.5: Comparison of Phonological/Phonetic and Morphological/Syntactic Disorders in Totally Blind and Partially-sighted Boys and Girls

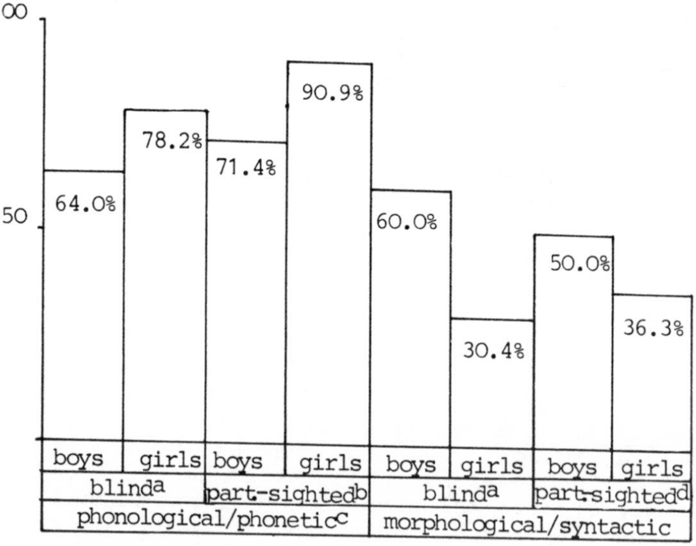

boys	girls	boys	girls	boys	girls	boys	girls
blind[a]		part-sighted[b]		blind[a]		part-sighted[d]	
phonological/phonetic[c]				morphological/syntactic			

Note: a. blind children (n=48)
Note: b. partially-sighted children (n=25)
Note: c. includes stammering of one or several sounds
Note: d. includes agrammatism and 'almost no speech'

33

When the phonological-phonetic and morpho-syntactic language abnormalities of children in KG I are compared with those of children in KG II, it appears that children in KG I make more articulatory mistakes but fewer structural (grammatical, syntactic, lexical and semantic) errors (see Figure 3.6). No mistakes in articulation were included from children listed under 'almost no speech'. This can easily be explained by the fact that the children of KG II had additional handicaps, particular mental handicaps, and therefore had greater problems with the formal properties of language.

Figure 3.6: Comparison of Phonological/Phonetic and Morphological/Syntactic Disorders amongst Boys and Girls of Kindergartens I and II.

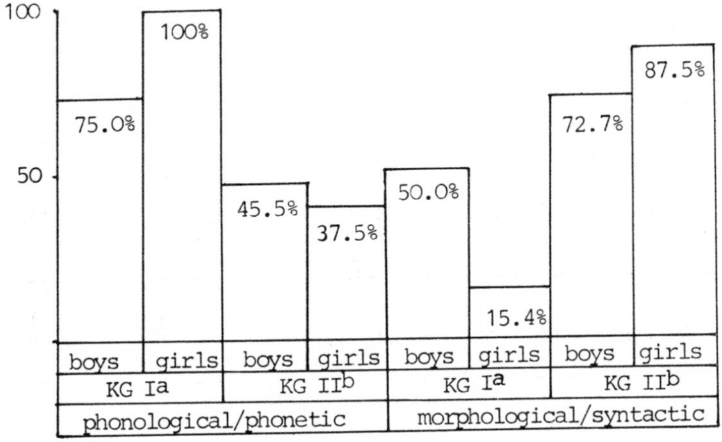

75.0%	100%	45.5%	37.5%	50.0%	15.4%	72.7%	87.5%
boys	girls	boys	girls	boys	girls	boys	girls
KG Ia		KG IIb		KG Ia		KG IIb	
phonological/phonetic				morphological/syntactic			

Note: a. KG I - boys (n=28), girls (n=26)
Note: b. KG II - boys (n=11), girls (n= 8)

Discussion of the Results

There are presumably several reasons for the large number of language abnormalities among blind and partially-sighted children at the Vienna School for the Blind (Figures 3.1 and 3.2). Firstly, one must recall all the dangers and problems which threaten the visually-handicapped child's mental and physical development, and therefore language development as well. These were discussed fully in the first section of this paper and were found in all areas of

language and communication.

The age of the children investigated (see Table 3.3) certainly contributes to the high incidence of language abnormalities. Many children of pre-school age have evidently not yet completed their language development. It is well known that sighted children also have far more language abnormalities at this age than later as school children, what Scholz (1970) calls "temporally influenced development".

The factor of social class seems also here to be relevant (see Table 3.4). It has been shown by some research, for example by Thimm (1977, pp. 79-80), that social class affects the rate of language development and skill in verbal expression. The children studied here belong predominantly to lower social groups. With the exception of one child, one could not expect pronounced verbal stimulation from the social environment. The two lower social groups show approximately the same incidence of language disorders.

Table 3.4: Categorization of Children in KG I and II according to Social Class

	Academic	Agricultural and Clerical Workers, Craftsmen	Unskilled
KG I (n = 71)	1 (1)[a]	56 (42)	14 (11)
KG II (n = 22)	0 (0)	13 (11)	9 (8)

Note: a. The figure in brackets refers to the number of language-disordered children.

An additional handicap to blindness seems to be the most important factor in explaining the high incidence of language abnormalities. As discussed above, children from KG II had relatively more abnormalities overall, especially in the dimensions of morphology, syntax, lexicon, semantics, and pragmatics (Figures 3.1, 3.2, 3.6), but fewer phonological problems. This can be attributed to the greater number of multiply-handicapped children in KG II. The most important of these handicaps were mental handicap and learning deficiencies, usually due to brain damage in early childhood, and pathological brain mutations with their corollary handicaps,

such as physical handicap, hearing disorders and motor disabilities. There was also one case each of diabetes and muscular dystrophy. Of the pre-school children from KG I 56.4 per cent (40 out of 71) were multiply-handicapped and from KG II 90.9 per cent (20 out of 22). Corroborating evidence can also be found in the literature. According to Graham (1968), almost half of all blind children who are multiply-handicapped are without language. It can be assumed with considerable certainty, that a large percentage of the remaining half have speech disorders.

Mental handicap correlates particularly strongly with language disorders. According to Young and Hawk (1955) approximately a quarter of the 53 children in their study had normal speech upon entering nursery school; on the other hand roughly the same number were without language, and over half had retarded or impaired speech. In 1968, Knolke reported that 19 out of 28 educationally-subnormal, blind children also had speech disorders. Among the subjects of our study, approximately 25 per cent of KG I and 86 per cent of KG II can be classified as educationally-subnormal or mentally-handicapped.

Educators of the blind point out that there is a constant increase of cerebral disabilities among blind pupils, which has critical consequences for the development of language. In this connection, Benesch (1974, p. 143) refers to the organic psycho-syndrome (defined by Bleuler) with its striking behavioural and motor disorders. According to the criteria set up by Benesch, signs of minimal cerebral dysfunction are already in evidence among nearly 50 per cent of the pupils at the Vienna Institute for the Blind and one can expect a further increase in the incidence of this brain disorder in the future. This necessarily implies a reconsideration of the educational consequences.

When there is a pronounced retardation in the development of pre-school children, one must always consider the possibility of the concurrence of cerebral disorders and social deficit. We were able to observe five-year-old children who were not yet toilet trained, had still not learned to walk properly, and refused solid food, because up to that point they had only received food of purée consistency or liquids (compare Rogow, 1972). Language development had not yet begun for these children, or had come to a standstill. The question should be raised here as to what extent one can make up for missed phases in development or compensate for

developmental disorders (Elstner, 1966, p. 35). Few of these children get the opportunity to enter educational institutions for normal children, and many turn out to be ineducable. The results cited earlier by Rogow (1973), Graham (1968), as well as Young and Hawk (1955) pertain to this issue.

The high proportion of disorders in language development leads one to ask whether the lack or limitation in spoken language is due to mental deficiency, or should be called a language disorder or language retardation[6] (from Leischner, 1967). Linck and Haberkamp (1976) and Kruse (1980) have contributed to the differential diagnosis of central disorders in language development. According to their work, a language disorder is now defined as organic damage of different brain functions or centres, whereas language retardation is defined as a "purely maturational problem in the language mechanism"[7] (Kruse, 1980, p. 208). Deafness and mental deficiency are not considered in the formulation of these definitions. A differentiated and specialized diagnosis at the Vienna Institute is not yet possible for several reasons. From the development we have observed over the past decades, however, we can conclude, that in approximately half the cases disorders in verbal communication are due to mental deficiency; approximately a third of the cases are to be classified as language disorders as defined above, and the remaining cases as language retardation problems.

When analysing the incidence of phonological-phonetic disorders and morpho-syntactic and lexical-semantic disorders between totally blind and partially-sighted children, it was found that, contrary to expectations, the totally blind did not show a generally higher incidence of disorders compared with the partially-sighted. This surprising result leads one to the conclusion that loss of vision is less of a crucial factor in causing a language disorder than the presence of an additional handicap or an unfavourable social background. Both of these factor have already been shown to be present in both the totally blind and partially-sighted. This conclusion is also supported by the data presented in Figure 3.6. This shows, in a comparison of the multiply-handicapped children (KG II) with the only visually-handicapped (KG I), that the multiply-handicapped have a higher number and more severe disorders especially in the areas of morphology, syntax, lexicon and semantics.

We see no contradiction in the fact that there

were fewer occurrences of articulatory mistakes among the severely handicapped children of KG II. This was because no phonological abnormalities were observed among the children without language from KG II, since no phonemic differentiation had begun yet. The children listed under 'almost no speech' could not rely on the spoken language alone for the purposes of communication. In the course of further linguistic development, however, more stammering is to be expected.

The prevalence of language abnormalities among children with partial vision (Figures 3.3, 3.4, 3.5) does not correspond to predictions made on the basis of previous studies (Häusler, 1968; Elstner, 1977). One can assume, however, as was indicated earlier, that this finding is not representative of the total population of blind and partially-sighted pupils, due to the small numbers and the negative selection with respect to additional handicaps. The partially-sighted pupils who entered the school at a later time had far fewer additional handicaps and therefore far fewer language disorders than the pre-school children.

We cannot explain the prevalence of language abnormalities among girls in KG II (Figure 3.2), the phonological-phonemic abnormalities of the children in KG I (Figures 3.5 and 3.6) or the morpho-syntactic abnormalities of the children in KG II (Figure 3.6), other than to attribute them to chance.

Figure 3.7: Causes of Difficulties in Verbal Communication in Visually-handicapped Pre-school Children

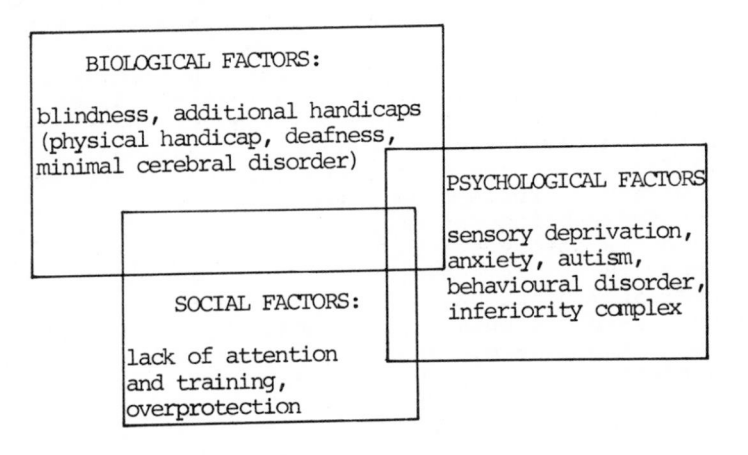

BIOLOGICAL FACTORS:

blindness, additional handicaps (physical handicap, deafness, minimal cerebral disorder)

PSYCHOLOGICAL FACTORS

sensory deprivation, anxiety, autism, behavioural disorder, inferiority complex

SOCIAL FACTORS:

lack of attention and training, overprotection

Although the different comparisons have produced no definite results, and it was not possible to conduct a statistical analysis, certain facts seem clear. Generalizing from these results, it can be said that children, as they enter pre-school institutions for the blind today, have comparatively more phonological-phonetic, morpho-syntactic, and lexical-semantic language abnormalities, as well as more difficulties with speech flow than sighted kindergarten children. The reasons are biological, mental and social in nature. These three factors overlap, as the preceding figure shows (see Figure 3.7).

Speech Therapy for the Visually-handicapped

To conclude this paper I would like to give a brief description of speech therapy work with the visually-handicapped child. On the whole it can be said that the general principles of speech therapy apply equally to the treatment of the visually-handicapped as to the treatment of the sighted (Elstner, 1971, p. 238). It is always an advantage to conduct therapy sessions in the environment where the child lives and plays, that is in his familiar physical and social environment.[8] The speech therapy then has the advantage of being "communicatively open" (Homburg, 1981, p. 273), that is, able to meet the wishes and needs of the child in the most natural way.

Training exercises for the various senses should accompany specifically language exercises, as has already been discussed in more detail (Elstner, 1971, p. 241 ff; Kiphard, 1972; Affolder et al., 1980). I have also published a collection of such exercises suitable for the visually-handicapped elsewhere (Elstner, 1972). It is important that everyone who has regular contact with the child be involved in such a programme to maximize the possibilities of improvement.

The exercises for the treatment of phonological and phonetic problems are also basically those used with sighted children. A clear diagnosis of the phoneme inventory has to be made, taking account of the age of the child, before therapy can begin (Scholz, 1970, p. 98). In order to introduce new sounds into the child's repertoire it is useful to proceed from characteristics of the sounds already known, what we have called the "deductive method" (Führing, Lettmayer, Elstner and Lang, 1981). Since there appears to be a need to improve auditory

perception (Lux, 1933; Elstner, 1955; Häusler, 1968), exercises to increase auditory attention and discrimination are used. Using the sense of touch, children follow movements of the lips and tongue, as well as perceive with the finger tip the size of mouth-opening appropriate for a particular articulation. These are possible compensatory exercises for the missing visual information (see Mills, Chapter 5).

In dealing with problems in the morpho-syntactic, semantic and pragmatic areas, it is important to refer to the stages of development in non-handicapped children, as has often been stated by other authors (eg. Miller and Yoder, 1971 quoted in Schiefelbusch and Lloyd, 1974, p. 543; Kubiak, 1979, p. 363). Emphasis has shifted within linguistics in the last decade from syntax to semantics and pragmatics. It is important that therapy also reflects the results in these areas (Ihssen, 1977, p. 171).

It must be stressed that no coherent description of acquisition in non-handicapped children is available for the speech therapist. With special reference to the visually-handicapped, a more complete analysis of the role of vision in language development is needed. Until such a description is available, the explanations offered for the high incidence of language disorders can only remain imprecise. Speech therapy must then also suffer from not having a clearly formulated basis for compensatory teaching.

NOTES

1. [Stimmen zu unterscheiden, aber sie kommen aus dem Unbekannten und kehren ins Unbekannte zurück.]
2. [Sprachverhalten wird von der Umgebung und/ oder dem Individium selbst als auffällig beurteilt, wenn es auf der phonologisch-artikulatorischen, morphologisch-syntaktischen oder lexikalisch-semantischen Ebene gegenüber den von sozialen Gruppen und Instanzen unterschiedlich formulierten Sprechnormen abweicht, wobei je nach Auffälligkeit des Sprachverhaltens neben der kompetenten Handlungsfähigkeit des betroffenen Individiums auch Beeinträchtigung seines Lernverhaltens in den Bereichen Kognition, Emotion, Psychomotorik und Soziabilität wahrscheinlich sind.]
3. Partially-sighted pupils can be instructed in the same way as sighted pupils, with the help of special teaching aids. They do not learn Braille.

4. [Konsekutive Verbildungen] These disabilities are the consequence of a primary handicap and are frequently psychological in nature.

5. KG I: For visually-handicapped children who would probably have otherwise received a normal education. KG II: For visually-handicapped children with additional, particularly mental, handicaps who would probably have nevertheless required a special education in the absence of blindness.

6. [SpEB - Sprachentwicklungsbehinderung], [SpEV - Sprachentwicklungsverzögerung]

7. [reine Reifungsstörung der Sprachanlage]

8. Since most (ca. 90%) visually-handicapped children live in residential schools, this would be in the living quarters of the family group.

Chapter 4.

SPEECH THERAPY FOR THE BLIND

Chris Schaner-Wolles

In the previous chapter Elstner provides an excellent opportunity for a person inexperienced in the field of blind-research, like myself, to gain insight into the problems involved in the physical, psychological and linguistic development of blind children, and their relation to the task of speech therapy.

The study which he presents covers all types of language problems which were present in pre-school children at a Viennese institute of education for blind children. In view of the extensive data sample and the large variety of problems dealt with, I will confine myself here to the discussion of a few of the more important points.

Mainly, I should like to emphasize the urgent need for linguistically and psycholinguistically based tools for diagnosis and analysis of pathological language development in children generally and that of blind children in particular. In the German speaking world at least, linguistics has not dealt with these problems in any satisfactory way. This affects not only Elstner's work, but is also a major stumbling block to the whole current practice of language therapy (see Dressler and Schaner-Wolles, 1981).

A well-founded diagnosis on a linguistic basis should draw up as complete a profile of all linguistic abilities of the child as possible. Such a general diagnosis requires a distinction to be made between the various linguistic levels, namely phonetics, phonology, morphology, syntax, semantics, lexicon and text, and for these to be correlated with different modalities, such as perception, imitation and production. Only after a complex analysis of all these levels will the nature and genesis of disorders become sufficiently clear to base an

42

adequate treatment on the insights gained into the specific features of the linguistic development of the handicapped child.

In practice however, disabilities at the phonetic level (disorders of articulation, fluency and voice production) are over-emphasized, whereas those disabilities at the other linguistic levels are still neglected, because of the lack of knowledge about structure, function and development of language (see Ihssen, 1978, p. 63). Elstner's work reflects the confusion between linguistic levels which is common in research into language disorders. For example, the distinction between speech and language disorders is not kept clear; a large number of so-called "language" or "phonological" disorders turn out on closer scrutiny to be at the phonetic level. Morpho-syntactic disorders are lumped together without any subdivisions; semantics and lexicon are touched upon unsystematically at best, while the textual level is neglected completely.

Since the population of Elstner's study is very heterogeneous - a feature to which I will return below, it seems worthwhile to check for deviant, delayed or "mixed" (Crystal, 1980, p. 127) language development. Does the development of a blind child differ in quality from normal language development with respect to the various linguistic abilities (Menyuk, 1964, 1969)? Hence, are the inferences drawn from comparison with the development of normal children necessarily fallacious? Or will the visually-handicapped child pass through - with a certain time-lag - the same stages of mental and linguistic development as the normal child (Lenneberg, 1967)? It seems that the search for the answers to these questions has been hampered by the lack of linguistically-based diagnostic tools and, for German at least, the lack of comparative data from language development of non-handicapped children (see Mills, forthcoming, for a review).

Unfortunately, the consequences for therapy are serious. In my opinion, it is impossible to work out a systematic and effective therapy programme without a clearly defined, detailed diagnosis. A therapy programme which is linguistically tailored to the individual child must be based on a diagnosis which establishes which aspects of the language abilities are delayed and which are deviant, and furthermore, the extent of deviance and delay. While, in the case of deviance, the programme has to focus on the specific characteristics of the language inventory of the individual child, in the case

of a delayed development, it is the acquisition
pattern of the normal child which has to be taken as
the basis for therapy.

Elstner seems to be intuitively aware of these
faults in speech therapy work. He mentions, for example, the frequent confusion of /m/ and /n/ in the
language of blind children, in contrast with sighted
children, and suggests an explanation. On the basis
of this explanation, he then tries to draw conclusions for speech therapy, which in this case could
not be inferred from experience with visually normal
children. He emphasizes the serious problems of
speech therapists in the area of morphology and syntax, as well as with respect to the lexical and semantic fields. He stresses the urgent need to work
out concrete principles in therapy work based on the
already existing vast body of theoretical literature, but for the individual therapist this is out
of the question (see Rieder, 1980, p. 4).

My contribution therefore is not so much intended to be a straight critical evaluation of
Elstner's work, but rather to be a plea for an interdisciplinary collaboration in research on pathological language development in children. The conference on which this volume is based, indicated
that the first steps in this direction are being
taken.

The point I should like to discuss finally is
not only crucial for the work under consideration,
but rather is a good illustration of how long the
road to cooperation still is, at least from an Aus-
trian point of view.

How reliable are the results of a study which
is based on a heterogeneous sample? The only property common to all subjects is, at worst, the fact
that they are all blind or partially-sighted. Brain
damage, mental retardation, or hearing impairment,
to mention just a few factors which certainly have
an impact on language development, could not be
checked in detail by Elstner before gathering his
data. This is the case simply by virtue of the fact
that, for whatever reason, a differentiated and
specialized medical and psychological diagnosis has
not yet been introduced at the Viennese Institute.

From my own experience with mentally-retarded
children, I am well aware that this situation is no
exception in Austria, nor, I presume, in many other
European countries. I wonder how a speech therapist
can do reasonable work under these circumstances: a
question therapists are increasingly asking themselves.

44

It is the task, and duty, of research workers in the medical, psychological and linguistic fields to make their findings accessible to those who wish to apply them, particularly in therapy work. The cooperation envisaged here has recently proved its value in research on aphasia (see Peuser, 1978). Interdisciplinary work such as this volume represents will hopefully bring us a good deal nearer to that goal!

Chapter 5.

ACQUISITION OF SPEECH SOUNDS IN THE VISUALLY-
HANDICAPPED CHILD

Anne E. Mills

THE ROLE OF VISUAL INFORMATION

The role of visual information, that is of the seen
articulatory movements, has not been the subject of
much research, although it has been known for a long
time that the seen articulation can improve comprehension when the acoustic conditions are bad. This
has been shown by O'Neill (1954) and by Sumby and
Pollack (1954) in perception experiments. Models of
speech perception therefore have not included visual
information but have been based on the processing of
auditory information related in some ways to articulatory movements.

The many studies which have investigated lip-
reading (for example Alich, 1960; Woodward and
Barber, 1960; Fisher, 1968; Walden et al., 1977)
have shown that the number of visually distinctive
sounds are smaller than the number of phonemes in a
particular language (called a "viseme" by Erber,
1974). This number is determined by several factors, for example the distinction between a voiced
and a voiceless sound does not appear to be visually
distinctive. The precision of the articulation and
the conditions under which the articulation is observed can also effect the number of distinctions
that are possible. The groups of consonants, based
primarily on the German phoneme repertoire, which
are visually distinctive under the most favourable
conditions are presented in Table 5.1.

It is not possible to describe the processing
of auditory information in detail here. What is
most important are the relationships between the
various acoustic parameters in the perception of
sounds. Miller and Nicely investigated the perception of sounds under different levels of white
noise. They found that the information necessary to

distinguish voiced from voiceless sounds and the information determining manner of articulation was
lost less quickly than the information determining
place of articulation.

Table 5.1: The Visual Groups of Consonants tested by Mills
and Thiem (1980)

Visual Group	Consonants[a]
1	b,m
2	v
3	ð
4	ʃ
5	l
6	r
7	z
8	d,g,n,ŋ,x,h

Note: a. Voicing is not relevant here.

Miller and Nicely wrote (1955, p. 352): "The place
of articulation, which was hardest to hear correctly
in our tests, is the easiest of the features to see
on a talker's lips. The other features are hard to
see but easy to hear."
     Visual and auditory information seem to comple-
ment one another. The exact interaction between the
two has not been the subject of much detailed investigation, although this topic has attracted interest
in recent years (Ewertsen and Nielsen, 1971; Dodd,
1977; McGurk and MacDonald, 1976, 1977; Summerfield,
1979; Mills and Thiem, 1980; McGurk and Buchanan,
1981). The results obtained by Dodd (1977) suggest
that visual information does not just support auditory information but plays an independent part in
perception. The results obtained by McGurk and
MacDonald (1977) also suggest this conclusion. They
presented adult subjects with a dubbed film in which
a speaker articulated syllables with the structure
consonant + vowel /ɑ/. The film was dubbed in such
a way that the articulatory movements of one syllable were presented with the sound of a different
syllable. The subjects frequently perceived illusions which did not agree in many instances with
either the seen or the heard syllable. For example

if /gɑ/ was presented visually and /bɑ/ auditorily, the subjects generally perceived /dɑ/ which is called a fusion. On the other hand, if they were presented with /bɑ/ visually and /gɑ/ auditorily, they most frequently perceived /bgɑ/, called a combination. On the basis of their results, McGurk and MacDonald formulated a manner-place hypothesis, since rejected, according to which the information as to the place of articulation is visual and the information as to the manner of articulation is auditory. This explanation however does not explain the two different types of illusion. According to this hypothesis the last case should lead to the perception of /b/ since this consonant is also a stop.

In a larger experiment including consonants which occur in German (Mills and Thiem, 1980) a greater range of consonants was tested in this way to see if a more exact explanation of the illusions could be found. According to the results of this experiment, four groups of consonants appeared to be visually distinctive in German (see Table 5.1), namely visual groups 1,2,3 and 4-8. In general the auditory information determined the voicing of the percept and the manner of articulation. The visual information determined the visual group of the percept. This still does not offer an explanation for the two different types of illusion, fusions and combinations. The perceived sound seems to depend on the articulatory possibilities which the visual picture allows as a whole. For example if a bilabial closure is presented visually (vis.gp.1) the lips are first closed then opened for the articulation of the vowel. As the lips open, they move through positions which match the articulation positions necessary for visual groups 2,3, and 4-8. When a sound from these groups is presented auditorily, it is possible to interpret the visual information as matching two different sounds, that is a combination. If the visual stimulus shows a greater lip opening than that necessary for the auditory stimulus then the perception of a combination is practically impossible. In the cases where the visual group contains a sound which has the same manner of articulation as the auditory stimulus, then a fusion is perceived.

These results suggest that the visual information determined to a very large extent what is perceived, in that an adjustment of the auditory information is more readily made than an adjustment of the visual information. This dominance implies that

the information from the auditory and visual modalities are compared with one another. A sound must be stored with its acoustic properties but also with the visual information about the articulatory movements. Models of speech perception must take visual information into account.

VISUAL INFORMATION IN THE ACQUISITION OF SPEECH SOUNDS

Under normal conditions of conversation visual information does not play such a critical part, firstly, because such discrepancies as were manipulated under experimental conditions are not possible and secondly because semantic and pragmatic information plays an important part in perception when words are involved. In the period of language acquisition in children, however, it is quite possible that visual information is more important than in adults. There is some evidence already to support this. In many diaries of child language development it is reported that the child around the age of six months watches mouth movements. Children often copy such movements without sounds (Scupin and Scupin, 1907). Wundt (1911) claimed this observation of mouth movements was critical in language development in that it formed the impulse to speak. An earlier study (Mills, 1978) with a sighted child (0;9) showed that the child used visual information in his imitations. The child tried to copy the different lip positions of the adult models.

From the hypothesis that sighted children use visual information in the acquisition of phonology follow certain predictions:

1. that sighted children will learn the articulatory movements that they can see more quickly and with less error than those that they cannot see.

2. that sighted children will make phonological substitutions within a visual group rather than across visual groups. The substitutions within a visual group will be made on the basis of other factors such as acoustic similarity. If a visual group has only a few members and these are not acoustically similar to one another, the sounds will not be substituted for one another.

3. that blind children will not be influenced in their phonological substitutions by visual groups but by other factors such as acoustic similarity. Substitutions will therefore be made across visual groups and a pattern will emerge which is different

from that of the sighted child.

Subjects and Method

To examine the accuracy of these predictions, a group of blind children are being studied in their early language development[1]. Here the analysed data from one blind child, Hanna, will be compared with the data from two sighted children. Hanna is a girl born of German parents. She is congenitally blind (Leber's tapetoretinal degeneration) with no apparent additional handicap. She has normal hearing and is well developed in motor and cognitive skills (well within the normal range). At the time of the recording of the data to be discussed here (1;9 to 2;1), she was just beginning to produce the first two-word utterances. The one sighted child, Joanna, is a girl of English parents. She is within the normal range in development, has normal hearing and was just beginning to produce two-word utterances at the time of recording, that is at the age of 1;6. The second sighted child, Amahl, is a boy of English father and Indian mother whose phonological development in English was described by Smith (1973). The data presented by Smith start around 2;2 since the boy began to speak late, at approximately 1;10.

The data collected from Hanna and Joanna consist of spontaneous utterances and elicited imitations of syllables with the structure consonant + vowel /ɑ/. Among the spontaneous utterances a distinction can be made between imitations of words occurring in the adult's previous utterance and productions which do not appear to have an immediate model. This distinction did not appear to have any effect on the data collected so that this distinction is not pursued. The data collected by Smith are predominantly spontaneous utterances and those considered here were collected between 2;2 and 3;0.

Elicited Imitations

The first comparison will be made between the elicited imitations of syllables from the blind child Hanna and the sighted child Joanna (see Table 5.2). The syllables are grouped according to the visual groups discussed earlier. Where it was not possible to elicit an imitation, a dash appears in the table. The data here are few since the imitation game was not always successful but in one instance they are of particular interest.

Table 5.2: Elicited Imitations of Syllables from One Blind Child (Hanna) and One Sighted Child (Joanna)

Visual Group	Model	Hanna	Joanna
1	b	b	b
	m	m/n/v	m
2	v	v	w
4-8	d	d/g	d/g
	g	g/d	-
	n	n	n
	s	-	j/g
	ʃ	ʃ/s/ç/θ	-
	l	l	l

    Hanna and Joanna both make errors in their imitations, mainly in substituting sounds within visual group 4-8. Hanna uses a sound from a different visual group in two instances: she produces, in imitation of /m/ (vis.gp.1) [n] (vis.gp.4-8) and [v] (vis.gp.2); in imitation of /ʃ/ she produces in one instance [θ] (vis.gp.3). Joanna makes substitutions within group 4-8 except for the substitution of [w] in imitation of /v/. This sound was not used in the illusion experiment which forms the basis of categorisation, since /w/ is not a phoneme of German. On the basis of Walden et al.'s results (1977) with English, it can be confused in a lip-reading task both with sounds of group 4-8 and group 2. It cannot therefore be clearly assigned to a visual group.

Spontaneous Utterances

More information is available from the spontaneous utterances. For the purposes of this analysis the initial consonants of the words produced were compared rather than the consonants occurring later in the word. Smith's data are used in this comparison. For the sake of brevity I will discuss the errors that occurred with visual groups 1 and 2 (see Tables 5.3 and 5.4). Firstly, the total number of target words beginning with a consonant from the visual group is listed for each child. Secondly, the number of words always produced with that consonant are listed. In the next two columns the substitutions

in these words are classified: where the consonant
was omitted and where the consonant was substituted
by a consonant from a different visual group. Errors in voicing were not classified as errors, so
that in visual groups 1 and 2 no substitutions
occurred within the visual groups. In the last
column all the other words produced by the child
were considered; the number of times a consonant
from visual groups 1 and 2 was substituted in these
words is listed. Errors where the first consonant
of a consonant cluster was omitted, such as /s/ in
/sm/, were not considered.

Looking at Table 5.3 first, which reports the
errors involving consonants from visual group 1, it
can be seen that the blind child makes more errors
across the visual groups. The figures from Smith's
data are presented for two periods since the errors
were concentrated in the first two months of observation. Even in this more restricted period the
number of errors involving substitutions across visual groups is still far smaller as a proportion of
the number of words involved than in the blind
child. If the actual errors are considered, the
difference between the sighted child and the blind
child becomes more marked. In every instance except
one, the sighted children's errors can be explained
by the influence of a consonant occurring later in
the word. For example, Amahl and Joanna produced
[berbu] for *table*, Amahl produced [bʌbə] for *rubber*,
[mɪbu] for *nipple*. The one exception is [maɪp] for
knife. Hanna's errors can only be explained in this
way in two instances. The other errors are different. She produced [deɪdi] for *Baby*, for example,
that is a vis.gp. 4-8 consonant is substituted for a
vis.gp.1 consonant; *tief* 'deep' was produced as
[pɪːf] (a vis.gp.1 consonant is substituted for a
consonant from gp.4-8), *weg* 'away' as [mɛp] and
fahren 'drive' as [pɑːl] (a vis.gp.1 consonant is
substituted for a vis.gp.2 consonant).

It could be argued that fewer errors are made
by the sighted children because these particular
individuals are more accurate phonetically. Smith's
data, since they are more extensive, were examined
to make a comparison of the productions of target
words beginning with /d/ and /t/ (vis.gp.4-8). Of
the 171 target words beginning with /d/ and /t/, 32
(19%) are produced with a different consonant (voicing errors are not considered). The main substitution was with [k] or [g] which are also from visual
group 4-8.

Table 5.3: Substitutions in Spontaneous Utterances from One Blind Child (Hanna) and Two Sighted Children (Joanna and Amahl) which involved Consonants from Visual Group 1 (/b/, /p/, /m/).

Child	Number of target words with initial vis.gp.1	Correct	Consonant omitted	vis.gp.1 substituted by different vis.gp.	vis.gp.1 substituted for different vis.gp.
Hanna	20	17	0	3	5 out of 95
Joanna	12	12	0	0	1 24
Amahl					
2;2-2;3	68	68	0	0	7 355
2;2-3;0	328	324	2	2	8 1400+

Table 5.4: Substitutions in Spontaneous Utterances from One Blind Child (Hanna) and Two Sighted Children (Joanna and Amahl) which involved Consonants from Visual Group 2 (/f/, /v/)

Child	Number of target words with initial vis.gp.2	Correct	Consonant omitted	vis.gp.2 substituted by different vis.gp.	vis.gp.2 substituted for different vis.gp.
Hanna	16	7	0	9	6 out of 99
Joanna	3	0	0	3 (all by /w/)	0 33
Amahl 2;2-3;0	96	64	0	32 (26 by /w/)	9 1600+

This number of errors is proportionally higher than the number of errors with /b/, /p/ and /m/, which suggests that Amahl is not generally accurate phonetically. This also supports prediction one, namely that sighted children will make fewer errors with the sounds which involve articulatory movements which can be seen than with those whose articulatory movements cannot be seen. Of the 13 words beginning with /d/ or /t/ which Hanna produced, three (23%) were produced with a different consonant, which indicates that she is not generally retarded in her phonological development.

Table 5.4 shows the substitutions involving consonants from visual group 2. A similar picture emerges. Again the blind child made a far greater number of errors across visual groups. The two sighted children, both English speakers it will be remembered, substituted /w/ in the majority of the cases. The status of /w/ is unclear in terms of its visual distinctiveness but, even if it is assumed to be distinct from visual group 2, the sighted children still make fewer substitutions across visual groups. In the nine errors produced by Amahl four words began with the morpheme *some* which was produced around the age 2;6 as [fʌm]. The other five substitutions were in words beginning with the cluster /sw/ which was produced as [f], for example *swing* as [fɪŋ]. The nine words can therefore be reduced to two rules, only one of which clearly involves a substitution across visual groups. Hanna's errors are again distinct, and are not clearly the results of any rules. In words beginning with /f/ or /v/, she produced for example [lʌs] for *Wasser* 'water', [haɪkə] for *weiter* 'further', [sɸlə] for *fühlen* 'feel'. /f/ was substituted in *Schuh* 'shoe' to produce [fuə], *Sack* 'sack' is [fʌk].

Discussion

Although the sample from the blind child is comparatively small, the evidence here is in support of the predictions made earlier. In support of prediction one, that is that sighted children will learn the articulatory movements that they can see with less error than those that they cannot see, Amahl made fewer errors in words beginning with /b/, /p/, and /m̈/ (vis.gp.1) than in words beginning with /d/ or /t/ (vis.gp.4-8) whose distinctive articulatory movements cannot be seen. The blind child made more substitutions across visual groups than the two sighted children and these substitutions did not

appear to be the result of any rule, such as assimilation, which was the case for the sighted children. From the evidence presented here the three predictions appear therefore to be upheld.

The question now remains to be asked what relevance this different pattern of substitutions has for the development of phonology and language in general for the blind child. In the case of Hanna, her general language development was within the normal range as far as structure and function were concerned, so that no overall effect could be observed. Her phonological development is retarded in comparison with that of the sighted child only in respect of those sounds which have an observable articulation, that is the sounds in visual groups 1 and 2. Her production of consonants which do not have clearly visible articulation however appears to be at the same level as the sighted children, so that she cannot be said to be generally phonetically retarded. From the evidence presented here, Hanna's different pattern of substitutions is not therefore to be classed either as retarded or deviant in the sense of a language disorder, but it is a different, marginally slower, developmental pattern. It is predicted that she will finally make use of acoustic information sufficiently to correct her substitutions and to conform to adult norms.

Considering Elstner's data (Chapter 3), it remains an interesting question, whether the different pattern of substitutions observed in Hanna could in itself lead to the development of different phonological rules and finally a language disorder. It would seem unlikely that this would result but, compounded with some other factors such as an additional handicap, it could well lead to a disordered phonology requiring therapy. Further research should throw light on this question.

NOTES

1.   This research project 'Die Rolle der visuellen Information beim Spracherwerb' is being conducted at the University of Tübingen and is funded by the Deutsche Forschungsgemeinschaft.

Chapter 6.

THE VISUAL AND AUDITORY MODALITIES IN PHONOLOGICAL ACQUISITION

Barbara Dodd

The results presented by Anne Mills in Chapter 5
demonstrate that speech perception involves not only
the processing of auditory cues, but also, if it is
available, visually perceived lip-read information.
This conclusion has now been reached by several researchers using different paradigms, and is true for
English and German (McGurk and MacDonald, 1976;
Dodd, 1977; Mills and Thiem, 1980). Mills' paper
raises two important issues. One is the role of
lip-read information in the acquisition of phonology; and the other is concerned with how lip-read information is coded for speech perception.

THE ROLE OF LIP-READ INFORMATION IN PHONOLOGICAL ACQUISITION

Teachers of profoundly deaf infants claim that instruction in lip-reading can usefully begin as early
as six weeks of age. If they are right, then very
small infants should be aware of lip movements i.e.
be able to extract some information by observing the
changing pattern of lip shapes. I attempted to test
this hypothesis (Dodd, 1979) by observing 10 to 16
week old infants' reaction to nursery rhymes presented with speech sounds and lip movements in-synchrony and out-of-synchrony.
    Twelve healthy, full-term infants, acted as
subjects. The babies were seated in an infant
chair, and their attention drawn to a mirror in
which they could see reflected the face of an experimenter who was inside a sound-proof box. The experimenter attracted the baby's attention by calling
the child's name and making noise. Once the baby
was attending to the in-synchrony speech in this
brief familiarization period, the experiment began.

Each experimental session lasted a minimum of four
minutes. During this time the experimenter recited
nursery rhymes, brightly, maintaining eye-contact
with the infant wherever possible. Every 60 seconds
the stimuli changed from being in-synchrony to being
out-of-synchrony or vice versa. The out-of-synchrony presentation was achieved by using a tape recorder delay, so that the auditory information arrived
at the loudspeaker behind the mirror 400 ms. after
it was actually spoken. Alternate infants began
with an out-of-synchrony presentation. Each infant
had two trials of each type of speech; each trial
was one minute long. Two observers, who had a good
view of the infant, pressed 'inattention buttons',
that were connected to a polygraph recorder, whenever the infants were not looking at the face, that
is, for example, when they were fretting, pulling
clothing over their heads, had their eyes closed.
The polygraph measured the time course of the experiment in seconds, the type of stimuli presented, and
the two observers' perception of the infants inattention. Agreement between observers was 95 per
cent.

Table 6.1: Percentage Inattention to in- and out-of-Synchrony
Presentation

Subject	In-synchrony	Out-of-synchrony
DC	20.3	50.4
MK	17.0	87.0
VH	6.5	25.1
JM	25.0	28.5
SB	5.4	26.9
MM	29.2	36.6
RH	2.9	1.0
DJ	6.6	43.8
JD	15.8	44.2
ZC	8.3	10.4
CW	34.0	29.9
AF	8.0	27.7
Mean	14.9	34.3

Source: Dodd (1979).

The results showed that infants attended signi-
cantly less to the out-of-synchrony presentation
than to the in-synchrony presentation (Wilcoxon T=5,
N=12, p<0.01). This finding was confirmed by the
fact that several infants became distressed during
the out-of-synchrony presentation. Thus it would
seem that infants as young as ten weeks of age are
aware when speech sounds and lip movements do not
match, even though they do not understand what is
being said. If it is not an innate ability, then it
is acquired very soon after birth.

One implication of the finding that lip-read
information can be processed in infancy, is that vision may play an important part in the acquisition
of speech perception and production abilities. The
obvious way of measuring the role of vision is to
study the development of blind infants.

The literature shows an increased incidence of
phonological disorders in the blind school-age population (see Elstner, Chapter 3). However, blindness
per se is not a sufficient condition for disordered
phonology, since most congenitally blind children
acquire a normal phonological system, though their
development may be slightly delayed. Therefore the
role of vision must be assessed in terms of differences in the developmental pattern of phonology between blind and sighted children.

Anne Mills' case study of a blind child has
provided some fascinating data which point to the
conclusion that normally sighted children often make
substitution errors from the same visually distinct
class of sounds, whereas blind children may maintain
the correct manner of articulation but tend to substitute a sound from a different place of articulation.

Some years ago, I collected language data on a
21-23 month-old little girl, Nicola, who had been
born without eyes, but who was otherwise normal. I
have therefore reanalysed the phonological data,
according to Mills, to see if it lends support to
her findings. Note that the subject's general language development was well within normal limits.

The phonological data analysed consisted of 100
words that could be unambiguously discerned from
tape recordings of Nicola's spontaneous speech.
These were compared, on a word for word basis, with
the phonological realizations of a normally sighted
little girl over the age range 17 to 27 months.
However, 61 words out of 100 were produced by the
sighted subject between 21 and 23 months of age, the
same age as Nicola at the time of data collection.

A summary of the data is shown in Table 6.2.

Table 6.2: Comparison of Blind and Sighted Children's Phonology

Response Frequency	Blind[a]	Sighted[a]
Pronounced correctly	42	19
Both children pronounced correctly	14	14
Both children made same error	32	32
Pronounced differently	54	54
Error Types (per cent)	Blind	Sighted
Substitution from same visual category e.g. [mɔl] *ball*	15.4	36.1
Substitution from different visual category e.g. [sɪp] *ship*	23.1	12.8
Cluster Reduction e.g. [bɛk] *block*	39.9	21.3
Deletion e.g. [ɪŋ] *sing*	24.6	29.8

Note: a. Number of words = 100.

The data show that the sighted child was more likely to substitute a sound from the same visual category, whereas the blind child was more likely to substitute a sound from a different visual category. The finding supports Mills' data, and indicates that sighted children do use lip-read cues as a source of information in planning their phonological output.

This is not surprising since lip-reading provides information about how to make a sound whereas an auditory stimulus merely provides an abstract target to aim at. Blind children should therefore be at a disadvantage in acquiring phonology, and this is reflected by reports of delayed phonological acquisition, and a high incidence of phonological disorders.

PROCESSING OF LIP-READ INFORMATION

The results presented by Mills show that lip-read information is important for normal development of phonology, and for speech perception. Thus heard

and seen speech perceptions must be integrated at some point in processing. The nature of the code in which they are combined has yet to be determined.

Three possible codes have been suggested. Lip-read information may be immediately recoded into a code derived from audition, and then processed as if heard rather than seen. MacDonald and McGurk (1978) suggest, on the other hand, that it is possible to modify the Motor Theory of speech perception (Liberman et al., 1967) to include visual information, that is lip-read perceptions could be processed in a code derived from articulatory feedback. However, evidence from studies of the lip-reading and phonological abilities of the pre-lingually profoundly deaf indicates that neither of these candidate codes is adequate.

The deaf can identify rhymes (O'Connor and Hermelin, 1978), match homophones (Dodd and Hermelin, 1977), develop a spoken phonological system (Oller and Kelly, 1974), convert lip-read nonsense words to graphemes (Dodd, 1980), primarily on the basis of lip-read inputs. In other words, the deaf can abstract a phonological code from lip-read information. An alternative candidate code, a non-modality specific phonological code, seems worth considering. Such a code would be capable of processing and combining speech information derived from audition, vision and proprioception (Dodd, 1980).

A sensory handicap, like deafness or blindness, would reduce the efficiency of the coding leading to disordered phonology, or abnormal developmental patterns. However, because of the non-modality specific nature of the code, neither handicap would preclude the acquisition of phonological skills.

Chapter 7.

BLIND CHILDREN'S LANGUAGE IS NOT "MEANINGLESS"[1]

Barbara Landau

THE NATURE OF THE HANDICAP

A central issue in the study of blind children's
language has been the extent and nature of their
handicap. It is usually assumed that the blind
child's experience lacks some essential component
or components that promote normal language learning,
and that this experiential deficit is reflected in
distortions of the language system. On first
thought, one might indeed assume that blindness must
have a wide range of devastating effects; for example, it is clearly more difficult to navigate
smoothly through space without vision, it is often
more difficult to determine the addressee in a conversation, etc. For the blind infant, the situation
could be worse yet, since he must learn about the
world without the benefit of rich visual information
specifying the shapes, sizes, and textures of objects, spatial layouts and their transformations
over movement, and socio-emotional communicative
signals from caretakers. Sensitive observers of
blind infants, notably Selma Fraiberg (1977) have
proposed that these deficits in information have
drastic consequences for the blind infant, resulting
in delayed object permanence, distorted emotional
relationships, and deviations in language. Yet it
is not so obvious to all that these proposed delays
and deficits are necessary consequences to blindness.
Consider the case of language learning by blind
children. The crucial theoretical question there
must be whether or not vision is in some principled
sense necessary for language learning. Three possible hypotheses come to mind. Firstly, based on
Bruner's (1974/5) analysis of the importance of gaze
in establishing mutual reference, one might wonder
whether or not blindness would impede this first

step in language learning. Secondly, Wexler and Culicover's (1980) work on learnability theory suggests that situational-interpretive input may be necessary to guarantee language learning under real time constraints. On this view, one might wonder whether or not blindness would reduce the availability of situational interpretations, and thereby reduce the availability of meaning-surface string pairings necessary for syntactic learning. Thirdly, one might wonder whether or not blindness could impair the development of concepts standing behind word meanings, thereby rendering blind children's language 'meaningless', even if well-formed.

This latter hypothesis seems particularly well-favoured in the literature, based on the following general rationale: where relevant experience is lacking, concepts cannot develop; and where concepts are lacking, word meanings cannot be learned. On one level, it has been claimed that a wide variety of concepts, hence word meanings, must be different for the blind than for the sighted child; it is often supposed that lack of vision means lack of many concepts. Specifically, various educators and psychologists have claimed that use of "visual terms" by the blind are 'verbalisms' - empty and meaningless for lack of supporting visual experience (Cutsforth, 1951; see Warren, 1977, for review). Yet, the evidence adduced for these claims has been limited, because of both flaws in methodology and lack of theoretical articulation. Most investigators have not attempted a serious discussion of what, exactly, could be lacking in the blind child's experience, nor how this lack could significantly interact with the learning process.

THE INVESTIGATION OF BLIND CHILDREN

For the past several years, we have been studying language learning in blind children, to assess the role of 'context' - carried by the sight of objects, properties, events, and scenes - in developing meanings (Landau, 1982; Landau and Gleitman, forthcoming). We have wondered whether, indeed, the function from sensory experience to language is so tight that variation in or absence of modality-specific input will lead to deviation and/or distortion in expressed meanings. Our specific questions have been: 1. How do blind children express early vocabulary of objects and events, and later predicate-argument structure (object-event relationships)?

2. In particular, what consequences does blindness have for the development of visual terminology? 3. Are usages of these words indeed empty?

Our three subjects have all been blind since birth, or shortly thereafter. Angie was a full-term baby, a victim of congenital deformation of the optic nerve, with some possible light perception in one eye. At her first interview (29 months old), she was already functioning at a sophisticated linguistic level, with mean length of utterance (MLU) 3.60. Angie's language was comparable to sighted subjects of the same linguistic level, to the extent it could be analyzed by the standard measures of expressed meanings.[2] The other two children were three and two-and-a-half months premature respectively, and were victims of Retrolental Fibroplasia. Kelli is totally blind; Carlo has some light perception. Both of these children were studied from onset of language through 42 months.

Language Onset
Onset of single words was at about 23 months for Kelli, and about 26 months for Carlo. These ages are uncorrected for prematurity, but even if corrected by three months, they still indicate a delay, relative to the sighted mean (14.2 months, Bayley Scales of Infant Development). A general initial delay for the blind subjects is corroborated by normative data on blind children from Norris, Spaulding, and Brodie (1957), although most of their subjects as well as Kelli and Carlo still fit within the normal range (10-23 months, Bayley Scales).

Expressed Meanings: Vocabulary and Predicate-argument Structure
Given the general onset delay, one might wonder whether blind subjects are deviant or different in what concepts they express, and what words are used to express them. Kelli's and Carlo's early vocabularies shown in Figure 7.3, are compared to sighted children studied by Nelson (1973). Kelli's sample was recorded between 23 and 28 months, and Carlo's between 26 and 29 months. Nelson's subjects were between 15 and 24 months when they achieved the 50-word level (mean: 19.75 months).

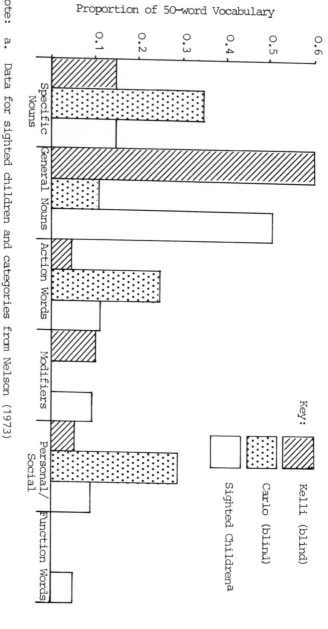

Figure 7.1: Early Vocabulary of Two Blind Subjects Compared to Sighted Children[a]

Note: a. Data for sighted children and categories from Nelson (1973)

Note that the early words expressed by both blind and sighted children are primarily objects and people (subsumed under specific and general nouns), and also include some action words (e.g. *go, up*) and personal-social words (*please, no,* etc.). Thus, despite the onset delay, there is no evidence from these data that blind children cannot express words for the concepts normally expressed by young children.

Next, consider the children's expressed meanings at a later language level, that is in early syntactic utterances. In Figures 7.2 and 7.3, the children's early multiple-word utterances are shown, compared to those of sighted children studied by Bloom and her colleagues, and using their coding system (Bloom, Lightbown and Hood, 1975).[3] In the earlier sample (Figure 7.2), both blind children express many action utterances (e.g. *Carlo open, Kelli eat*) and many locative actions (where the goal of movement was a change in location, e.g. *put in tape*). There are somewhat fewer locative states (where there is no movement effected, e.g. *Mommy sit,* when the mother is in her chair), states (expressions of wants or needs, e.g. *Carlo want cookie, Kelli sick*), attributes (e.g. *big truck*), and comments on the existence, negation, and recurrence of objects and events (e.g. *a dolly, no dolly, more dolly*). Note that Carlo shows fewer types of expressed relations than Kelli or Bloom et al.'s subjects. But in the later sample (Figure 7.3), both blind children express semantic relations covering all the categories.

These data suggest that knowledge of language is not diminished by blindness. Blind children do talk about objects and their locations in space, actions, and events, and do so in just the same way as sighted children at the same linguistic level.

However, some might still believe that the blind child is handicapped in language, choosing stronger examples to demonstrate this deficiency. The argument could be made that blind children can talk about objects and events since, after all, they can touch objects, and they can hear some events occurring. Yet their handicap exists since they do not have as much first-hand sensory experience with visual aspects of the world. This lack of experience must have some consequence: blind children can never know the meanings of words like *red* and *look* and *picture,* that refer to the visual world.

Figure 7.2: Early Sample of Semantic-syntactic Relations Expressed by Two Blind Subjects Compared to Sighted Children[a]

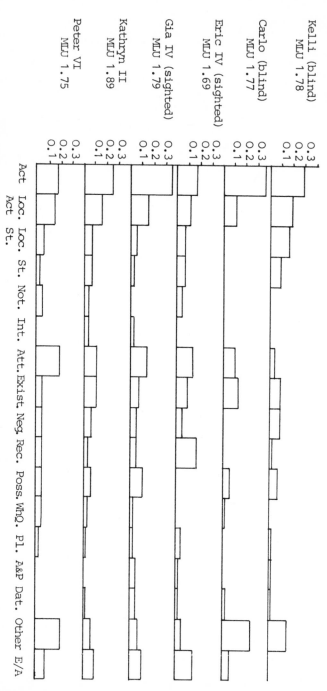

Note: a. Data for sighted children and categories taken from Bloom, Lightbown and Hood (1975)

Figure 7.3: Later Sample of Semantic-syntactic Relations Expressed by Two Blind Subjects Compared to Sighted Children[a]

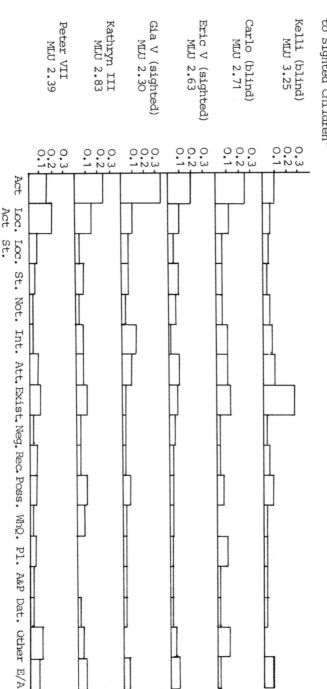

Note: a. Data for sighted children and categories from Bloom, Lightbown and Hood (1975)

Such a claim is certainly worth testing, although informally, we know that blind adults do use language to refer to visual aspects of the world - for example, they do say *look* and *see*. Defenders of the deficiency notion emphasize that the use of such visual words by the blind is 'verbalism', or empty and meaningless usage. Yet the evidence for such a claim is merely a handful of studies, using methods such as word association, elicitation of imagery, and the semantic differential (see Warren, 1977, for review). These methods are at best highly indirect and at worst irrelevant in assessing the blind person's meanings (or lack thereof) for visual terms.

What would be convincing evidence that verbalisms are a function of deficient concepts? One possibility would be data demonstrating that use of the terms reflects an impoverished, inconsistent, or bizarre concept. For example, it might be that the blind person uses the work *look* to mean simultaneously "scratch the left elbow" and "buy milk at the corner store". This would certainly be bizarre, and would provide some preliminary evidence that sighted concepts are not constructable without relevant sensory input.

Is there any such evidence? We do not believe that there is, but much more importantly we have evidence that is altogether counter to the belief that use of visual terms by the blind is semantically empty. Our evidence is in the form of intensive observation and experimentation on one of our totally blind subjects.

Use of Sighted Terminology for Haptic Activity

Kelli began using the visual term *see* when she was 28 months old, approximately the same age at which sighted children begin to use verbs of perception. From the beginning, Kelli's use of the word *see* was far from meaningless. To people around her, she seemed to use the word when she wished to touch some object; and she was satisfied when her request to "see" something was followed by letting her touch it. This behaviour suggested that visual verbs like *see* and *look* meant "touch" to Kelli.

Indeed, it did seem to mean "touch", for in a first series of experiments, we asked Kelli to *Look up*, and she responded by straining her hands upwards above her head, as if to reach some object. This is hardly the response of a sighted child to the same command, and it is not even the response of a sighted child deprived of vision by blindfolding. When

four sighted control subjects were blindfolded and asked to *Look up*, they responded by tilting their heads upwards, as if genuinely trying to look at some object. So Kelli's use of *look* was surely different from the sighted child's use. Yet it was not bizarre, since her method of contact is manual; nor was it inconsistent, for when she was asked to *Look down, Look in front of you, Look behind you, Look over here*, or *Look over there*, she responded with the spatially appropriate movement of her hands, "looking down" by touching the floor, "looking behind" by touching the floor in back of her, etc. Note, too, that Kelli did not understand the word *look* in its broader sense, that is, either to mean "perceive in general", or to mean "understand", as we sometimes use the term (e.g. *I see*, or *Look at what you're saying*). Rather, *look* was differentiated from other verbs of perception; for when Kelli was asked to taste something, she put it to her mouth, and when asked to listen to something, she put it to her ear, or simply quieted, attending to some expected sound. But when asked to look at or touch some object, Kelli reached out, contacting the target object with her hands.

If Kelli's meaning for *look* was synonymous with *touch,* this would have been an interesting finding. But as it turned out, her meaning was not simply identical to *touch*; rather, *look* seemed to mean "perceptually explore with the hands", while *touch* meant "simply contact with the hands". We discovered this during a long series of queries to Kelli, starting with the command *Touch (some object) but don't look*. To this potentially contradictory command, Kelli merely laid her hands on the object, without exploring it. When she was told to *Look, but don't touch (some object),* she either explored manually (the normal response to *Look*), or responded with confusion. This initial set of behaviours suggested the distinction between *look* (perceptually explore) and *touch* (merely contact), which we then documented in a series of 30 commands, modifying the verbs *look* and *touch* along four dimensions: spatial, intensity, temporal, and instrument of perception. For example, we asked Kelli to *Look* or *Touch under/here/behind; Look* or *Touch real hard/gently/ real good; Look* or *Touch once/not yet; Look* or *Touch with your finger/foot/nose/mouth/ear.*

On many of these commands, Kelli differentiated *look* from *touch,* always "looking" by exploring and manipulating, and "touching" by coming into manual contact in a non-exploratory way. For example, if

asked to *Look behind you*, she searched for an object behind her; but if asked to *Touch behind you*, she touched her back. When asked to *Look real hard* at some object, she rubbed it up and down, but when asked to *Touch it real hard*, she would bang the object with her hand, or scratch it with her fingers. When asked to *Look with your nose* or *Look with your mouth*, she performed the appropriate modality-specific behaviour, for example, bringing the object to her mouth as if to taste, or to her nose as if to smell. But when asked to *Touch with your nose* or *Touch with your mouth*, she bent down, and pressed that part of her body to the object.

So it seems that Kelli did use *look* in an internally consistent and meaningful fashion, to mean "explore with the hands", and contrastively with *touch* which meant "simply contact the object". At least from this evidence, it again seems that the blind child does use words like *look* and *see* in a meaningful fashion.

Learning that *Look/See* Means "Explore with the Hands"

How could Kelli have learned these words? First, of course, the words have been used by people around her. In fact, the simplest explanation of Kelli's usage would be that she has directly imitated usage by some model, say her mother. If Kelli's mother used the words *look* and *see* in just those contexts when Kelli was manually exploring an object, then perhaps the fact that Kelli developed a meaning for these words is not at all mysterious.

But it is indeed mysterious, since Kelli's mother did not use *see* and *look* exclusively to refer to Kelli's tactial-haptic perception of objects. Rather, her mother used the words in many other ways as well: to mean "visually perceive" to her sighted child, Kelli's younger sibling; as a simile (e.g. *Kelli, you look like a kangaroo*); and in contexts where Kelli could not possibly look at an object with her hands (e.g. when Kelli was in another room). And it is important to note that Kelli's mother herself was quite unaware of her child's meaning, for she was astonished when Kelli's arms flew upwards to the command *Look up*. She was astonished, for she and her husband had taught Kelli to tilt her head upwards to the command *Look up*, and downwards to the command *Look down*.[4] Kelli's novel response to these commands in the experimental situation is a powerful demonstration that some abstract representation of

the word *look* was guiding her response (rather than some memorized routine).

How, then, did Kelli learn these meanings for *look, see,* and *touch*? First, note that many natural languages carry the same distinction for verbs of perception as the one that Kelli made: the distinction between the exploratory mode of perceiving, and the non-exploratory mode. For example, in English, we have such a distinction for verbs of vision, with *look* versus *see*; and for verbs of audition, with *listen* versus *hear*.[5] Further, we have the expression *to set eyes on,* meaning "merely direct one's eyes towards", as in *I never even set eyes on him, much less knew him well.* Wasco (an American Indian language) also encodes this distinction for visual verbs, but more succinctly than does English: there are two monomorphemic items, one corresponding to the English phrase "set eyes on" ("put two eyes on"), and one to the phrase "visually explore". For tactual verbs, French encodes the distinction, with the verbs *tâter* meaning "palpate", and *toucher,* meaning "merely come into contact with the hand". These similarities across languages in encoding the exploratory/non-exploratory distinction for perception verbs provide insight into how Kelli came to make the distinction between *look* and *touch*. In particular, it seems to be a fact about humans that it is important to distinguish between these two modes of perception. Language, reflecting this distinction, often (though not always) separates the two modes by allotting a different basic word to each. Kelli, of course, is human, so it is presumably important to her to differentiate between active and non-active perception with her dominant modality - the tactile-haptic system. Kelli was not provided with a direct linguistic reflex of this distinction in English; so she must have commandeered the work *look*, an otherwise stranded word, and used it to mean "haptically explore".

Learning that *Look/See* Means "Perceive with the Eyes"

Let us now return to the notion of handicap in blind children's language. Earlier, we mentioned that a favoured hypothesis about the source of this handicap is the notion that sensory experience furnishes the building blocks of concepts, which, in turn, stand behind word meanings. In the extreme, it has seemed self-evident to some that the blind child could never know what was meant by visual terms.

Yet Kelli has furnished us with evidence forcing rejection of this claim for a handicap induced by blindness: as we have just seen, the use of words *look* and *see* by this blind child is far from meaningless. Rather, the child has created her own meaning, one which is internally consistent, and far from bizarre, as it is a distinction normally carried by natural languages. One might say, at this point, that it is the strictly visual use of visual words that is the handicap; for example, Kelli could never come to know what it means for a sighted person to "see".

But we also have evidence that she has this knowledge, too. We have documented Kelli's comprehension and production of visual verbs referring to the activity of sighted persons; and we have found that Kelli knows well that vision conforms to the laws of Euclidean geometry. She knows that sighted poeple need to have objects correctly oriented in space to be able to see them, that sighted people cannot see through barriers (although they can hear through barriers), that large objects must be displayed differently from small objects for sighted people to see them at a distance, that certain spatial operations on an object can make it invisible and that these are different from the operations that can make an object inaudible (see Landau, 1982; Landau and Gleitman, forthcoming, for details).

Is Kelli then aware that sighted people are different from blind people? We believe she does have a growing awareness of what her own blindness means, since we have observed her commenting on occasion *Mommy, because I can't see?* or *Because I'm blind?*. These comments occur in contexts that are deeply related to her experience as a blind person, for example, when she is puzzled that others can "see" photographs, or airplanes, or birds in the sky. It seems that Kelli's knowledge of blindness grows with her knowledge of the meanings of sighted words.

Kelli's knowledge of the sighted meanings for visual terms, although surprising, can be understood. Clearly, the environment provides a basis for learning from experience. Kelli has learned about vision through her knowledge of space (see Landau, Gleitman and Spelke, 1981), and through language, since there was never any parental restriction on the use of sighted words to her. So, for example, several occurrences of her mother saying *I can't see you* when occupying various locations relative to Kelli might suffice for the inference that

sighted people can see only if there are no barriers
(and, if the object is correctly oriented). Or, the
similarities in linguistic structures over different
verbs of perception might suffice to indicate there
is an active-stative distinction for the visual mode
of perceiving. For example, the distinction between
active-stative modes is carried by syntactic context. That is, to the question *What are you doing?*, one might reply *I am looking/listening*, but
less plausibly, **I am seeing/hearing*. In short,
various kinds of knowledge have entered into Kelli's
learning, by inference, that sighted *look* and *see*
mean something quite different from her own, haptic
look and *see*.

CONCLUSIONS

Kelli has demonstrated that blindness need not lead
to deficits in language learning; and indeed, that
rich representational capacity underlies even use
and understanding of visual terminology. Why, then,
did anyone ever think of visual language by the
blind as a deficit? Most likely, because of underlying theories about human learning, in particular,
about how we come to have the concepts we do, and
how we proceed to learn the language that expresses
those concepts. The notion that the blind child
cannot learn to use visual terms meaningfully comes
close to the heart of the classical Empiricist programme on issues of concept acquisition. The radical Empiricist view of these issues is, roughly,
that the primitive base of concepts is occasioned as
a direct reflex of the sensory apparatus; complex
concepts are built out of these primitives. Where
there is no sensory reflex for a primitive - e.g.
colours for the blind man - there should be no concept (see Fodor, 1981, for discussion of the pit-
falls of this programme). John Locke, representing
this view, wrote:

> I think it will be granted easily, that if a
> child were kept in a place where he never saw
> other but black and white till he were a man,
> he would have no more ideas of scarlet or
> green, than he that from his childhood never
> tasted an oyster, or a pineapple, has of those
> particular relishes. (Locke, 1690)

According to this view, then, the blind child
has no appropriate sensory reflex for terms

referring to visual experience, and further, does not have the materials necessary for learning the terms (see Fodor's discussion of the differences here between the empiricist and rationalist programmes). The layman's or educator's version of this theory finds the blind child deficient when he uses visual terms, and discourages such use.

Without the case of the blind child, we might speculate that this view is too simple; for we do learn words like *truth, liberty,* and *humanitarian,* whose meanings (or meaning features, if one could decompose them) seem far removed from any specific sensory experience. But the case of the blind child forces us to modify the radical empiricist view of concept and word-learning, by providing one simple and direct example: the blind child learns concepts for *look* and *see*, even though she cannot look or see. Her knowledge is gained through experience, but the relevant experience is far more complex than a direct reflex of the sensorium. Rather, the experience is the subtle product of a complex interaction between internal biases about the assignment of words to concepts, and knowledge from other conceptual domains - such as space and language.

Finally, if we adhered to a direct and simple view of the relationship between the sensorium and language, we would overlook important theoretical and practical issues. First, we would obscure theoretically important facts about the nature of human language learning, for example, the internal biases that bring a learner like Kelli to create a lexical distinction between exploratory and non-exploratory tactile-haptic perception. And second, practically, we would be misdirected in our suggestions for parental treatment of blind children. We might suggest, as Cutsforth did decades ago, that the blind child be discouraged from using visual terminology, lest it lead to "loose thinking". Could use of visual words lead to "loose thinking"? I believe Kelli has shown us that the opposite is true: for free use of visual terms has allowed Kelli both to make crucial linguistic distinction for her own means of perceiving, and to understand what is meant by the other, visual, means of perceiving. Ultimately, this knowledge can lead Kelli to profound insights into the nature of her own blindness.

NOTES

1. All of the work reported in this paper was done jointly with Lila R. Gleitman. I wish to thank

her for her extensive theoretical insights and involvement in every aspect of the project. In addition, I thank her for copious comments on previous drafts of this paper. Thanks also go to Dr. Gilberto Pereira and Ms. Anne Farren of Children's Hospital of Philadelphia for locating subjects, and to Lenora Knapp and Marcia Glicksman for analyzing data. This work was supported by a Social and Behavioral Sciences Research Grant from the National Foundation - March of Dimes to Lila R. Gleitman, and a National Research Service Award from the National Institute of Mental Health to Barbara Landau.

2. The measures we used were developed by Nelson (1973) to characterize early vocabulary, and by Bloom, Lightbown and Hood (1975) to characterize semantic-syntactic relations in early syntactic utterances. Therefore, the measures were more appropriate for analyzing language at an earlier growth point than Angie's level at her first interview.

3. Note that these comparisons are again between the sighted and blind children at the same linguistic level (MLU). As with previous analyses, the blind children are older than (delayed relative to) their sighted controls.

4. Her parents had taught Kelli to *Look up and look down* with appropriate (sighted) head movements in the context of a nursery song, simply as part of the action accompanying the song.

5. The contrast between *touch* and *feel* is ambiguous, since *feel* can be used either in an exploratory or a non-exploratory way, for example, *Feel this fabric*, versus *Can you feel* (i.e. sense) *that?*.

Chapter 8.

MEANING IN LANGUAGE ACQUISITION

Paul Werth

MEANING IN PSYCHOLINGUISTICS

In recent years, psycholinguistic studies of meaning
have tended to make certain simplifying assumptions
about their object of study: (1) that meaning re-
sides in, is the property of, words; (2) that the
analysis of word-meaning should be componential,
i.e. composed of minimal elements, arranged in some
order; (3) that the acquisition of word-meanings is
gradual, i.e. component by component, rather than
holistic; (4) that the relationships between components are actually acquired by way of a procedure
(which may be based on logical or ontological knowledge).
   Consider the following quotation from Clark and
Clark (1977, p. 509):

   When children acquire the meaning of a word,
   they construct an entry for it in their mental
   lexicon. They start off with a very simple entry containing only a few of the components
   relevant to its use by an adult. And as they
   learn more about its meaning and how it contrasts with other words, they may add further
   components and, if necessary, discard irrelevant ones. Eventually, their entry comes to
   coincide with the adult entry.

   This by now orthodox view embraces points (1-3)
above; for point (4), see Clark and Clark (1977, p.
439 ff) and Miller and Johnson-Laird (1976, p. 122
ff, and passim). From the more purely linguistic
point of view, we should clearly want to know more
about (a) the "adult entry", i.e. what components it
contains, and how they are arranged, and (b), more
generally, what is the nature of these components,

77

whether they come from a set of universal semantic primes, or a language-specific set, and what are the restrictions on their possible combination and structural-hierarchical arrangement.

In the previous chapter Barbara Landau was concerned with the sensory language of sensorially-deprived children. She provides us with a method and some data which bear upon two areas of great importance in the study of human cognitive development: (1) the relationship between the linguistic-conceptual systems of the blind and those of the sighted; (2) the nature of the meanings acquired by children, and where and how they originate.

Underlying the first area is a tradition of received beliefs and fallacies about the language of the blind, while beneath the second area are the various competing theories of meaning. The re-examination of the first area requires us to apply what we know about language and cognition in general in the explanation of new facts emerging from the study of the language of the blind, enabling us to preserve or modify one or another theory in the second area.

THE MEANING OF PERCEPTION VERBS

Let us begin by quoting Miller and Johnson-Laird (1976, p. 585) on verbs of perception, (including those studied by Landau): "*Perceive*... is a predicate that denotes the process involved when an internal representation of the external world is constructed out of information from the receptors."

Assuming this definition to be substantially correct, the implementation of the process poses some interesting empirical questions, two of which Landau concentrates upon: (1) What do blind children mean (do) when they employ visual terms? (2) How do they construct such meanings, and particularly, from what input?

Visual Meanings in the Blind

Landau argues that the *see/look* modality has been translated - for at least one child - into the *touch* modality. It seems clear that in very broad terms, this is correct, for Kelli substitutes manual exploration for visual examination. But there are some disturbing weaknesses both in her experimental design (casting some doubts on the reliability of her findings), and in her linguistic assumptions

(revealing a crucial gap in her experiments).
First, (a perhaps unavoidable problem for most
small-scale psycholinguistic research), there is a
risk with small numbers of subjects that any findings are, at best, merely anecdotal, and at worst,
actually misleading because they may accidentally be
unrepresentative. Notice that the philosophy of
science meta-argument appealing to existential generalization (i.e. that the existence of a single
case is sufficient to require the modification of a
general theory), does not serve to generalize the
behaviour of Kelli to all blind children or, for example, Washoe-behaviour to all chimpanzees. Rather,
it applies when the single case is a case of some
phenomenon which the theory is directly or indirect-
ly setting out to explain, for instance, in a theory
of grammatical sentence-types, a sentence-token of
the language under scrutiny. But we have to ask:
what counts as a 'sentence token' here? In fact, a
'single' sentence-token represents not a single case
of linguistic behaviour, for example one utterance
of one speaker on a single occasion, but a set of
<u>recurrent behaviour patterns across a group of</u>
<u>speakers</u>. What makes it 'acceptable', both to
speakers and as a datum for such a theory, is (a)
that it is recurrent, and (b) that it is generalized
across a 'dialect'-group. In other words, the
'single' sentence represents a large number of utterances or judgments, and not merely one. Kelli's
behaviour with *see* and *look* certainly seems to be
recurrent, but we have no evidence yet that it is
generalized. Without amassing a lot of corrobora-
tive evidence from a statistically-significant number of other cases, we have no real indication that
this is anything more than Kelli-behaviour (which
could be originally random, and reinforced by some
chance contingency; cf., for example, the 'private
languages' of twins).
    Fortunately, such a defect is easily remedied.
More worryingly, however, there are occasional weaknesses in Landau's experimental design, particularly
when it comes to controlling for variables. A small
example: to test whether Kelli understood the difference between *touch* and *look*, Landau gave the
child such instructions as *Touch but don't look at*
some object; Kelli then duly distinguished between
the two verbs. The problem is that the very instruction itself invites a contrast, and thus ob-
scures the difference between a natural distinction
and a forced opposition; any child at all asked to
Touch but don't feel or *Look but don't see*, or

Talk but don't speak would be likely to force some differentiation, just to be compliant.

Another methodological problem arises out of the inevitable play element in this kind of research with small children. Given that comprehension or intended meaning are typically investigated via non-linguistic response (usually involving the manipulation of toys), what counts as a successful (or meaningful or useful) answer might vary from a thorough-going performance of an appropriate activity right through to a more or less reduced iconic representation of it (e.g. *Taste the dolly* - Kelli puts the doll to her lips). Just as a young subject might be anxious to please this nice adult who brings interesting toys, and spends time playing with her, so might the researcher run the risk of 'over-interpreting' the responses. Especially if her data consist of the iconic type of response, the researcher is in danger of misrepresenting her results by making possibly untenable assumptions based on inadequately-specified responses.

CONSTRUCTION OF MEANINGS, AND THEIR INPUT

The input of a semantic system such as Kelli's for *see/look*, argues Landau, must come from (a) spatial knowledge and (b) syntactic contexts. She makes some interesting observations in support of these, but does not adduce any really strong evidence or theoretical argument to back them up. We must consider, therefore, what would constitute such evidence or argumentation.

Spatial Knowledge
For the sighted speaker, the verb *touch* in its primary sense requires the object to be within reach of the bodily extremities; *feel* as a haptic verb implies substantial bodily contact; *look* and *see*, on the other hand, suggest non-contact. All - unlike *hear* and *smell* - imply the absence of some kind of intervening material. For Kelli, though, *touch, feel, look* and *see* are all contact-verbs when transitive (*Look at the doll*), but not necessarily so when intransitive (*Look behind you*). Given this distinction, it would be interesting to find out something more about the precise meaning for Kelli of the intransitive cases: what exactly does *Look behind you* mean when translated into the touch modality? I suspect that for a sighted speaker it is

a more precise instruction than it is for Kelli
(viz. *Turn through a semicircle until your eyes are*
± *180° from their present position,* as against *Scan
the hemispherical space to your rear*). I suggest
this for no better reason than the sheer physical
difference between the optic and the haptic modalities. Spatial knowledge presumably derives from all
sensory inputs together: relatively close space
from all senses; further space from vision primarily, less from hearing. But the most important faculty for the acquisition of any knowledge is of
course the symbolic-conceptual - what we may call
'central processing', (or perhaps, specifically,
"the ability to reason" (Miller, 1967, p. 15) or
"deductive information processing" (George, 1970, p.
140) or even "logical competence" (Wason and
Johnson-Laird, 1972, p. 41)). Central processing,
we may hypothesize, is not only responsible for the
interpretation and classification of sense-percepts,
it is also responsible for building up a conceptualization from the various sources at its disposal:
the senses, memory, the (developing) language system, and particularly its semantic component, together with problem-solving and decision-making
skills. In the absence of any visual input, presumably the most important source of spatial information for the blind child must be language (Landau
certainly seems to assume this). Let us therefore
consider the role of linguistic context for these
perception verbs.

Syntactic Context

Landau suggests that the active/stative distinction
in English, between *look* and *see*, or *listen* and
hear, for example, would have become obvious to
Kelli from the usage of those around her, illustrated in Example 1.

Example 1. (What are you doing?) I am $\begin{cases} \text{looking} \\ \text{listening} \end{cases}$

*I am $\begin{cases} \text{seeing} \\ \text{hearing} \end{cases}$

There are several syntactic points to make here.
First, note that Example 1 as presented is rather
rare and highly context-dependent, as in Examples 2a
and 2b.

Example 2. (a) (Can I help you sir?) No, it's al-
right, I'm just looking.
(b) Will you please be quiet. I'm
listening.

In such contexts, where the object of attention is
either non-specific or obvious, the normally transitive verbs *look* and *listen* may occur without an
overt object. From Example 1 alone, a blind child
would be able to infer no more than the information
that looking and listening are activities, while
seeing and hearing are not. In their normal contexts, however, *look* and *listen* take objects (with
prepositions). Second, it is a well-known teaching
point about English that the verbs of "inert perception" (Leech, 1971) do not accept the continuous aspect, so that *see* and *hear* in Example 1 would be
discounted on those grounds anyway. However, and
thirdly, even without the continuous aspect, *see* and
hear, being verbs of "inert" perception, are not
usually possible responses to questions with *do*:

Example 3. (What did he do?) *He $\begin{Bmatrix} \text{saw} \\ \text{heard} \end{Bmatrix}$ the
accident.

Moreover, there are several other possible contexts which Kelli could have been exposed to:

Example 4. <u>V + Adj.</u>
John $\begin{Bmatrix} \text{looked} \\ \text{felt} \\ {}^*\text{saw} \\ {}^*\text{touched} \end{Bmatrix}$ amazed, silly,
tired...

Example 5. <u>V + Prep. phr.</u>
Myrtle $\begin{Bmatrix} \text{looked} \\ \text{felt} \\ \text{saw} \\ {}^*\text{touched} \end{Bmatrix}$ over, through,
around... the room.

Example 6. <u>V + THAT-comp. S</u>
Oedipus $\begin{Bmatrix} {}^*\text{looked} \\ \text{felt} \\ \text{saw} \\ {}^*\text{touched} \end{Bmatrix}$ that his mother was
ready.

Example 7.   <u>V + Obj. + Manner adv.</u>

James $\begin{Bmatrix} \text{looked at} \\ \text{felt} \\ *\text{saw} \\ \text{touched} \end{Bmatrix}$ the newspaper care-fully.

Example 8.   <u>V + IF/WHETHER-comp. S</u>

Go and $\begin{Bmatrix} \text{look} \\ \text{feel} \\ \text{see} \\ *\text{touch} \end{Bmatrix}$ if the bed is dry.

We can see from these examples that there is not a great deal of apparent consistency here: on the face of it, *look* variously behaves like each of the others, and enters into almost all the possible combinations. However, this apparent confusion is at least partially resolved when we look at the regular semantic distinctions which operate within the category of perception verbs as set out in Table 8.1.

Table 8.1:   The Semantic Distinctions between Verbs of Perception

Sense (Perceive)	Sense Receptor Activity	Sensory Exploration	Appear To Senses
See	Set eyes on	Look at[a]	Look
Feel_S	Touch	Feel over[a]	Feel_A
Hear_S	Attend to	Listen to[a]	Sound
Smell_S	Sniff at	Smell_E	Smell_A
Taste_S	Savour	Taste_E	Taste_A

Note: a.   or another preposition

We can see from Table 8.1 that the four forms in the *see* and *hear* modalities are distinct from each other (taking the prepositions to be part of the form). *Feel, smell* and *taste*, however, are more ambiguous - nevertheless, if they are differentiated by indices, as has been done in the table, we can go a long way towards sorting out the contextual chaos.

Thus, Example 1 has the sensory exploration meaning, Example 4 has the appear-to-the-senses meaning, and Example 6 has the perceive meaning. Examples 5, 7 and 8, though, are still mixed. We can explain Example 7 in this way: the manner adverb is sensitive not to this particular categorial set, but to the active/stative distinction (cf. Ross, 1972), which brings the sense-receptor meaning and the sensory-exploration meaning together as activities. Example 8 is somewhat harder: it seems to me that the basic meaning here is 'perceive' and the non-perception verbs (*look*, and perhaps *feel* too) are portmanteau-forms:

Example 9. Go and $\begin{bmatrix} \text{look at} \\ \text{feel over} \end{bmatrix}$ the bed and $\begin{bmatrix} \text{see} \\ \text{feel} \end{bmatrix}$ if it is dry.

In Example 9 the first parenthesis encloses exploration-verbs, and the second, perceive-verbs. This leaves as our only remaining mystery, Example 5: basically, this seems to be the sensory exploration meaning (the preposition performing an important role here), though it evidently allows of a more receptive sense with *see*. Of the other perceive-verbs, *hear* also has an occasional prepositional use as in Example 10.

Example 10. Evan heard through my explanations in silence.

The question remains, however: are there sufficient surface clues to enable these meanings to be distinguished from each other? Given the evidence that we have examined so far, it seems doubtful that there are. But this is as true for sighted learners as for blind ones: in fact, how does anybody learn to distinguish these meanings? Presumably, given that all speakers can correctly differentiate them, the cues must be more diverse and subtle than we have so far accounted for, and there is no particular reason to suppose that lack of visual cues provides any special difficulty.

However, Table 8.1 does reveal a glaring deficiency in Landau's argument. She strongly implies that, for Kelli, *look (at)* has ousted some of the area of meaning which for sighted people is occupied by the word *touch*: such that *look* has come to mean "explore", while *touch* now means "degraded contact But this is not in fact the case: *touch* never normally bears an exploratory or even a perceive sense.

As Table 8.1 shows, it is exclusively used for sense-receptor activity, i.e. it normally means something like "contact with the hand". The appropriate exploratory verb in the *touch*-modality is thus not *touch*, but *feel(over)*. But not one of Landau's experiments has apparently sought to investigate the meaning of *feel* for Kelli, and its relationship for her with *look*. What would Kelli have made of the instruction - perfectly coherent to a sighted person - *Feel over but don't look at the doll*? In fact, in the light of a systematic table such as Table 8.1, it would seem advisable for Landau to carry out a more extensive programme of testing <u>all</u> the oppositions involved.

To these suggestions, I think it would be helpful to add another. Perhaps with somewhat older children, it would be interesting to study how a blind learner deals with the meaning of more specific vision verbs such as *watch, stare, peep, peek, glimpse, glance, notice* and *glare*. These add further distinctions, not all of which would be directly perceivable by the blind child (e.g. both *watch* and *stare* suggest intentionality and prolonged duration, and the latter adds social impropriety; *glimpse* suggests the object is partly hidden, while *peep* suggests the perceiver is partly hidden, and so on). Would such distinctions be evident to, or difficult for, the blind child?

IMPLICATIONS

I now come to a more general discussion of the implications of Landau's paper. One of the notions which she quite rightly castigates is that of "meaningless language" or "empty verbalisms". She demonstrates that one blind child's visual language is not "empty". But is the notion of "empty verbalism" even coherent, even notwithstanding Kelli's example? Clearly, there are possible interpretations of the expression which make sense: the mere 'parroting' of unknown languages might be one such. But it would perhaps be more precise to call that a 'vocalism' rather than a 'verbalism', since the latter implies linguistic status for the utterance, and I find it dubious that something devoid of meaning <u>for the speaker</u> can be accorded linguistic status. Natural language certainly contains morphs which are "empty" in the sense that they have only syntactic function while lacking semantic content (e.g. *do* in questions and negatives, expletive *it* and *there*).

It is also of course possible for speakers to employ words of whose meaning they have not the foggiest notion (though they will characteristically know a great deal about their syntactic and even collocational behaviour). But morphs and words do not exclusively make up language; in fact, they are largely artefacts of analysis. In the terms we are examining, "language" and "verbalisms" refer to spoken utterances, necessarily. Utterances, unlike sentences or propositions, are real-world phenomena whose meanings are governed not by truth-conditions, but by relevance-conditions (cf. Grice, 1975; Werth, 1981; Wilson and Sperber, 1981). Thus, even in the case of a speaker deliberately violating the relevance-condition by including fictitious words in his utterance (like the comedian Stanley Unwin, for example), the utterance as a whole will still bear pragmatic, or contextual, meaning, even if this is only the implicature that the speaker is being deliberately unhelpful, or facetious. But this is unconventional behaviour, of course, even if it is interpretable. In the case of sensorially-deprived children such as Kelli, however, that sort of choice can still be made. The question of linguistic deficit, though, has arisen for areas of linguistic behaviour where it is assumed no such choice is possible; specifically, it seems to be assumed that a sightless person lacks experience for that area of conceptualization, and therefore cannot employ visual language other than "emptily". But this seems to be based on a fallacious premise, namely, that the input to the conceptualization of a given sense-experience is necessarily and exclusively the evidence afforded by that particular sense-modality: thus, goes this theory, a blind child has no input at all to visual conceptualization, and hence his visual language will be "empty". But consider again Miller and Johnson-Laird's definition of perception, given above. Let us assume, with them, that although there are five sensory input systems (sight, sound, taste, smell and touch), they all feed into a single perceptual system (our "central processor"). If this is so, we can then hypothesize that a child deficient in any of the input systems will nevertheless still be able to construct some sort of model of the world in his conceptual system, using evidence from his non-defective inputs (in which there may even be compensatory development). It seems that Kelli has been able to do something of this kind; but to test the hypothesis properly, we obviously need much more information from deaf and other

sensorially-handicapped children.

Moreover, if the hypothesis is true, a further interesting question arises: can we predict which sensory system will substitute for a given defective one? In Kelli's case, we can see that sight and touch have been related through a common concern with external form. Furthermore, Kelli's substitutions can only be possible where it is external form which is under consideration. Asked to look at colours or images or non-discrete phenomena, such as sunsets, Kelli would clearly be unable to comply, using touch or any other non-defective sense. But touch is not in fact the only conceivable modality which could be substituted for vision. With modern technology, such as the adapted sonar for the blind, one can imagine a sight-vocabulary using terms derived from an auditory one. For the deaf, loudness might be interpretable in terms of size or proximity (spatial systems), or via intensity of light or colour (visual systems).

To conclude, I will try to answer the question: is Kelli's language "deficient"? In the sense of "containing a meaningless set of visual terms", the answer is clearly that it is not deficient. But I must nevertheless say that we should not allow ourselves to get carried away by the discovery that *look* for Kelli has a regular and coherent meaning. The sad fact is, that the language of Kelli and children like her is <u>inevitably</u> deficient in at least these ways: (a) spatially: while it seems clear that Kelli has been able to construct some model of the world from her other senses plus deductive powers, nevertheless it is reasonably obvious that any such model will be incomplete and distorted (in ways systematically different from the individual distortions made by sighted children); and (b) lexically: for instance, though Kelli has at least partially substituted *see/look* for *touch/feel* etc., we must still ask what has become of the existing distinction between *see/look* and *touch/feel*. My guess would be that for Kelli it is there, but in a dormant way. She has a set of haptic meanings for both modalities so that for most purposes she will treat them as synonyms. However, if pressed, she has been able to construct some sort of second-hand conceptualization of vision which she can refer to. Obviously, though, it cannot be as full or detailed as that of a sighted child, and she will usually ignore a sighted distinction which, for her, is unproductive. Nevertheless, at this point, we may begin to wonder exactly how far-reaching the effect of

such a handicap is on concept-formation, anyway,
given that only a certain proportion of our conceptual store is formed through direct perception, and
even that has to go through central processing, including memory, reasoning etc. The remainder comes
from secondary experiences, mainly linguistic, and
for blind and sighted people alike, the resulting
concepts will most probably be incomplete, distorted
and false. The difference is that for blind people
there is an area of experience which can never be
detailed at first hand - but given that so much of
human language is non-visual (abstract, mental, emotional, "displaced" - cf. Hockett, 1960), we may
perhaps take comfort in the realization that blindness may not be an overwhelming handicap at the conceptual level, at least.

Chapter 9.

REFERENTIAL DEVELOPMENT IN BLIND CHILDREN[1]

Randa Mulford

INTRODUCTION

Of the several functions of language that a child
must master on his way to becoming a fluent adult
speaker, the referential function is one of the most
basic and one of the earliest to emerge during development. By the "referential function" is intended a speaker's ability uniquely and unambiguously to
identify for a listener the entity or entities being
talked about. The development of reference has been
a topic of considerable interest among language acquisition researchers in recent years. It has been
approached from a variety of perspectives, for example, by developmental semanticists (e.g. Nelson,
1973; Bowerman, 1978; Clark, 1979), pragmatists
(e.g. Bates, 1976; Atkinson, 1979; Ochs,
Schieffelin and Platt, 1979), psychologists (e.g.
Piaget, 1951; Bruner, 1975), and theoretical linguists (e.g. Halliday, 1975a; Lyons, 1975). These
researchers and others have traced aspects of the
development of linguistic reference from its pre-
linguistic roots through the mastery of complicated
and subtly differentiated referring expressions. Of
course, there is still much to be learned about many
details of referential development, but its general
outlines have become clear.
     For a number of reasons, the development of
reference is a particularly appropriate topic on
which to focus an investigation of blind children's
language. First of all, knowledge of the 'normal'
course of development in this area is relatively detailed. This puts researchers in a favourable position when trying to formulate specific bases for
comparing language acquisition in blind and sighted
populations. While gross measure of language development in the two groups (e.g. Norris, Spaulding and

Brodie, 1957; Fraiberg, 1977) have generally shown
few differences, more detailed comparisons of particular aspects of development (e.g. Rowland, 1980;
Mulford, 1981) suggest that there are indeed differences, some more striking than others, in the course
and rate of language acquisition for blind and
sighted children. If comparative studies are based
on well-documented aspects of normal development,
then it is more likely that comparisons can be made
that are sufficiently fine-grained to reveal the
subtle differences, or perhaps the similarities, between the two populations.

A second motivation for considering referential
development is that there is good reason to expect
blind children to face particular challenges in this
area. Accounts of sighted children's development
suggest that vision contributes in several significant ways to the growth of the referential capacity.
It might, therefore, be expected that visually-impaired children will encounter difficulties at various points in development where the role of vision
appears to be crucial. The second part of this paper will be devoted to trying to anticipate the
kinds of problems blind children may encounter in
learning to refer successfully and to illustrating
both some of the problems and some of their solutions with evidence from the existing literature on
language development in the blind.

Finally, the topic of referential development
is one in which two major lines of current research
on blind children's language, mother-child communication and semantic development, converge nicely.
As will become clear below, learning to refer successfully involves both taking into account and
manipulating aspects of the communication situation
and using linguistically appropriate referring expressions. These are precisely areas where much
previous and ongoing work on blind children's language has focussed. It therefore seems useful to
make explicit some of the links that exist between
lines of research which, at first glance, might seem
to be only vaguely related.

A FORMULA FOR ESTABLISHING REFERENCE

Before taking up the referential function from a
developmental perspective, it is necessary to consider what is involved for any given "act of reference" to be successful. Imagine the following situation: a speaker (A) wants to convey to an

addressee (B) that a particular object, say, a pencil, is broken. To convey this message, it is not enough for A to sit alone in his room and say *B, the pencil is broken*. Nor is it enough for A to enter a room where B is engaged in conversation with someone else and to say *It's broken*. Even if A takes B aside, looks him straight in the eye and says *It's broken* or *The pencil is broken*, it is still quite likely that B will not be able to figure out what A is talking about. The referent is unclear and the referring act is unsuccessful. More conversation will be necessary before A can get his message across to B.

Here is a 'formula' for how to refer successfully to some entity X, like the pencil in the example above. It is based on similar schemas proposed by Martin Atkinson, Eleanor Ochs and Bambi Schieffelin (see especially Keenan and Schieffelin, 1976; Atkinson, 1979; Ochs et al., 1979). It involves the following five steps or (self-)instructions to the speaker:

1. Assess whether the listener is paying attention to you.
2. If the listener is not attending to you, do something to get his attention.
3. Assess whether the listener is attending to the referent X.
4. If the listener is not attending to X, do something to direct his attention to it.
 - (Repeat steps 3 to 4 until the listener is attending to X)
5. Refer to X with a sufficiently definite, unambiguous referring expression.

In the hypothetical situations sketched above, the speaker A violated this formula in various ways. In speaking to someone who was not there, he failed to assess adequately the listener's attention. Even when he was in the same room with the speaker, he at first failed to gain B's attention before beginning to talk. When he succeeded in securing B's attention to himself, he failed to make sure that the referent object (the pencil) was also in B's attention. He further failed to use explicit enough referring expressions. Thus B was unable to interpret what particular object A had in mind when he used the word *it* or the phrase *the pencil*. A speaker must comply with all five steps of the referring formula before a given act of reference can be succesful.

There are many things a speaker can do to assure that the listener is paying attention to him
and to the potential referent. In practice these
two goals of attracting and directing the listener's
attention are very often accomplished simultaneously. Ochs et al. suggest a number of strategies,
both verbal and non-verbal strategies, that speakers
typically use to accomplish these goals. (L refers
to the listener and X to the referent entity.)

Non-verbal	Verbal
- initiate eye contact with L	- name L (vocative)
- move toward L	- name X (use some referring expression)
- touch L	- use greeting term (e.g. *Hi!*)
- point at X	- use deictic pronoun or adverb (e.g. *there, that*)
- look at X	- use expressive particle (e.g. *Uh-oh, Ow!*)
- touch X	- use locating device (e.g. *Look at X*)
- reach for X	- ask a question (e.g. *What's that?*)
- show X to L	- use a prosodic device (e.g. whine, change speech volume or register)
- give X to L	

The strategies that a speaker uses to attract
attention to himself are probably primarily determined by the social and/or physical situation. For
example, touching the listener may only be appropriate in an informal context, or when making noise
(e.g. by saying the addressee's name) would be undesirable. Strategies used for directing attention
to the referent, however, are highly dependent on
its physical location relative to the speaker-listener dyad. To return to the hypothetical situation
discussed above, the means that speaker A can use to
assure listener B's attention to the pencil in question will depend largely on whether the pencil is in
fact on the scene. If it is physically present,
then A has several options. For instance, he can
point at, look at, or hold up the pencil and then
say *It's broken*, assuming that B will be able to relate the gesture and the pronoun. Or he can use,
instead of a gesture, some verbal device, for example a definite referring expression, to pick out the
pencil. So A might say *Do you see the yellow pencil
lying on my desk?* and then add *It's broken*, thus
creating a linguistic link between the pronoun and

the object it refers to. Or the speaker can combine
both verbal and non-verbal devices to bring the pencil to B's attention. For example, he can hold up
the pencil, saying *See this pencil?*. Then he can go
on to complete his message *It's broken*. Certainly
this combining of strategies is very common in normal conversation when the referent object is physically present.

If, however, the pencil is not physically present at the time A wants to convey his message to B,
then the only means he has of identifying the referent are verbal. Non-verbal strategies like pointing,
touching or showing can only be used to draw attention to aspects of the physical environment, not to
referents which exist only in memory or in shared
knowledge. A is limited to saying something like *Do
you remember the pencil I bought when we were shop-
ping yesterday? Well, it's broken*. He must bring
the referent to B's attention by introducing it into
the conversation, in other words, by using language
only. This kind of reference to an entity not present in the 'here-and-now' of the speech context has
been called "displaced reference". The capacity for
displaced reference is one of the defining properties of human language.

Whether a speaker intends reference to the
'here-and-now' or to a more remote context, he is
obliged to use a linguistically appropriate referring expression or the referential act will be unsuccessful. The speaker who, for example, points at
a pencil and says *The crayon is broken* will certainly confuse his listener. Even saying *It is broken*
in the same circumstances may not be precise enough,
as the speaker could be intending the pencil as a
whole or only some smaller part of it (e.g. the
eraser). Successful reference requires the use of a
referring expression which is sufficiently explicit
to allow the listener to uniquely and unambiguously
identify what the speaker is talking about. The
linguistic and extra-linguistic conditions determining what is "sufficiently explicit" in any given
speech context may be very complex; they will not be
taken up further here. Every language user has,
however, undoubtedly had many experiences where, as
a listener, he has had to ask for clarification of a
referent or, as a speaker, he has had to make his
reference clearer. Thus this kind of referential
failure is certainly very familiar.

The formula for establishing reference outlined
here represents steps that any speaker must take
whenever he intends to refer. As was pointed out

above, in the course of actual conversation, many of
the "steps" can be and often are accomplished simultaneously, with speakers and listeners continually
assessing and directing each other's foci of attention within the physical and verbal contexts. (For
a more complete discussion of reference in discourse, see Keenan and Schieffelin, 1976; Ochs et
al., 1979.) The particular referring expressions
the conversational participants use are also highly
determined by the entire discourse context.

NORMAL DEVELOPMENT OF THE REFERENTIAL FUNCTION

The sequence of steps within a referential act also
reflects in interesting ways the typical developmental sequence as a child masters the referential
function of language. Research with sighted children shows that the development of reference proceeds along the general path to be outlined below.

Attracting Attention to Self
Infants become adept at attracting attention to
themselves considerably before they begin to talk.
At first their success at drawing attention to themselves is quite unintentional. They cry, smile,
gurgle and vocalize in reaction to internal or external stimuli, but their actions frequently have
the effect of attracting the attention of those a-
round them. Later, beginning around nine months,
infants start to make deliberate efforts to attract
the attention of others (Bates, Camaioni and
Volterra, 1975). They use basically the same repertoire of behaviours which has been successful in
eliciting notice unintentionally, but now they may
initiate the crying, vocalizing, smiling, etc. and
persist in the behaviour until they are satisfied
that someone is attending to them. Attracting attention to self, then, is developmentally one of the
earliest steps in learning to refer.

Assessing the Listener's Focus of Attention
How infants learn to assess other people's foci of
attention has perhaps been examined in less detail
than other aspects of pre-referential and referential development. It is clear, however, that from
an early age babies are sensitive to others' direction of gaze. They will look in the same direction
as someone else from about four months of age

(Bruner, 1975). Even before this, they seem to recognize making eye contact as a sign of mutual attention. Although vision seems to play a primary
role in assessing attention, infants also learn to
recognize and accept auditory proof of attention,
for example, adult imitations or other reinforce-
ments of the baby's vocalizations. Infants also undoubtedly recognize very early that touching, holding and other tactile exchanges may be signs of attention. Typically adults will show their attention
to the infant with a combination of signals, e.g.
vocalizing, gazing and touching simultaneously.

Directing Attention to External Referents
Shortly after infants have become successful at attracting attention to themselves, they begin to try
to direct others' attention to objects and people
outside themselves. Again, deliberate attention-
directing seems to have its roots in the baby's unintentional activities. For example, infants may
mouth, bang, vocalize at or look at objects in their
own explorations of them; adults may then treat the
infants' actions as deliberate attempts to bring the
object to adult attention. Intentional attention-
directing begins to appear when the infant is about
ten months old. Initially it draws upon the earlier
repertoire of object behaviour. Then some specifically attention-directing behaviours begin to
emerge, for example, showing an object and communicative pointing. These gestures come to be combined
with vocalizations during the pre-linguistic period.
Children may be motivated to combine vocalization,
and later language, with gestures as they become
aware that in some situations gestures alone are not
enough. If, for instance, the other person is not
looking at you, it is impossible to attract or direct his attention by pointing alone.
     As the first words begin to appear, they are
very often superimposed on attention-getting and
-directing gestures. One of the earliest items in
the vocabulary of most infants is some kind of
deictic or "attention-directing" word (e.g. *that,
there, look,* or some baby variant of these). It is
invariably accompanied by pointing or some other
gesture (see further Nelson, 1973; Carter, 1978;
Atkinson, 1979). Infants also come to use other
words, for example, the names of people and objects,
with these gestures; ultimately they are able to use
the verbal devices alone to draw attention. Typically, however, gestures continue to be used along

with language in many situations (Pechmann and
Deutsch, 1980).

Early Development of Referential Language

A baby's first uses of language with referential in-
tent may not be very accurate. A one- or two-year
old has, after all, only a limited vocabulary and
typically uses the words he has with meanings that
do not exactly correspond to the conventional meanings of the adult language. When, for example, a
child says *dog* to indicate a cat, horse or other
animal, he is not using the referring expression
very accurately. Semantic development is a gradual
process and such errors of meaning are very common
in early child language (Bowerman, 1978; Clark,
1979). Other more subtle problems in learning to
use the full range of referring expressions of the
adult language continue to plague the language-
learning child well into his school years (see, for
example, Karmiloff-Smith, 1979). Complete mastery
of the accurate use of referring expressions con-
tinues for many years, probably as long as a speaker
is learning new vocabulary.

Development of Displaced Reference

The child's first uses of verbal devices for reference are very strongly tied to the immediate speech
context, to the 'here-and-now'. Referring expressions are first used to indicate aspects of the per-
ceptible physical surroundings, to name people, objects, actions and properties that are on the spot.
First attempts at displaced reference generally appear from about age 18 months and are initially limited to the immediate past (i.e. comments about what
has just happened) or to the child's intentions for
the immediate future. Generally early displaced
references are triggered by some aspect of the current situation (Sachs, 1977). The capacity to talk
about more distant places and times depends crucial-
ly on the child's ability to use language alone,
without the support of non-verbal attentional strat-
gies, to make clear for the listener what he is
talking about. Children under about three years of
age are not very adept at displaced reference, especially when the listener is not a familiar person.
They are still very dependent on the non-verbal context to support their referential acts and are still
mastering those verbal devices which specifically
signal intention to refer to another time or place,

such as tense markers or phrases like *Do you remember...?* (Ochs et al., 1979). They are also not very good at assessing the listeners' knowledge of non-immediate situations and thus make many assumptions about other people's abilities to figure out what they mean.

POTENTIAL PROBLEMS FOR THE DEVELOPMENT OF REFERENCE IN BLIND CHILDREN

Clearly, the development of reference, as we understand it so far, is a very complex and drawn-out process. Let us turn now to the particular challenges blind children may face in mastering the referential function. At each step of the referring act, problems are likely to confront a blind speaker. Some of these problems, and some of the solutions that blind speakers might exploit, can be illustrated with examples from naturalistic speech samples collected during a longitudinal study of the language of three blind children. The subjects of this research were three totally congenitally blind boys between the ages of five and six. All were considered to be 'successful' blind children by the adults who worked with them. Two, Robert and Joshua, were identical twins whose blindness was due to retrolental fibroplasia (RLF). The third one, Alex, had Leber's amaurosis, a genetic retinal disorder. None had any other diagnosed sensory or central nervous system impairments. The children were recorded in various settings, but primarily in their pre-school or kindergarten classrooms or at home. The children and the data collection methods have been described in more detail elsewhere (Mulford, 1981). In the following dialogues, SC indicates a sighted child. Where more than one adult is involved, identity is indicated by a numerical subscript.

Assessing the Listener's Attention to the Speaker

Unless the blind child is already participating in a conversation with someone, he may have trouble determining whether his intended addressee is listening to him (Examples 1-2) or whether the person he wants to talk to is even present at all (Example 3).

Example 1. Joshua is walking across the classroom to a table where Adult$_1$ is sitting. In his path is another table where Adult$_2$

97

Example 1.   is seated. Joshua doesn't know Adult$_2$
(cont'd)   and hasn't been aware of her presence.

       Adult$_1$: *Over here, Joshua. Careful.*
                You're gonna run into the table
                with Mrs. Edwards. [=Adult$_2$]
       Joshua: [to Adult$_2$] *Where's (your)*
                car? [Adult$_2$ doesn't answer]
       Adult$_1$: *Say "Hi, Mrs. Edwards".*

Example 2.   While walking to the kindergarten class-
            room, Robert and Adult$_1$ have been talk-
            ing about asking Adult$_2$'s permission to
            go to the parking lot to see Adult$_1$'s
            car. They enter the kindergarten class-
            room, where Adult$_2$ is seated at a table
            at the opposite end of the room, out of
            earshot.

       Robert: *Becky* [=Adult$_2$], *could I see*
                Randa's [=Adult$_1$] *car, please?*
       Adult$_1$: *Becky's at the - way at the*
                other side of the room. (You)
                have to go down there (to
                where she is).

Example 3.   Robert, Joshua, Adult$_1$, and Adult$_2$ are
            seated at a small table. The boys have
            been playing 'the object game' together;
            Robert is now playing alone while the
            others observe. Mike, a high school
            student who often comes as a teacher's
            aid, is absent.

       Joshua: *(Mike), are you doing the ob-*
                jects with Robert?
       Adult$_1$: [not understanding who Joshua
                intends to address] *Yep, we're*
                watching him. O.K.?
       Joshua: *Mike?*
       Adult$_1$: *Mike's not here today.*

Knowing that the intended addressee is physically
present (e.g. touching the child or making noise) is
no guarantee that he is paying attention. Even if
the blind child has been conversing with another
person, he may have a hard time assessing whether
the listener's attention has shifted to someone or
something else, since he cannot rely on visual cues
to the listener's continuing attention. For example, the listener may be looking elsewhere (Example
4) or may have moved out of earshot.

Example 4. Adult₁ and Adult₂ have been talking with
            Alex about changing cars. Then they
            switch to consulting a map together.
            Alex: [to ?] (*Er-*)*um-am I going in
                   your car?* [being ignored] *Am I?
                   Am I?*
            Alex is apparently unaware that the
            adults' attention has shifted to the
            map.

It seems likely that blind speakers rely heavily on
auditory or verbal confirmation of listener attention and actively try to elicit such confirmation.

<u>Attracting the Listener's Attention to the Speaker</u>
As discussed above, many of the sighted child's earliest attention-getting strategies are non-verbal.
Some of the most effective of these, such as initiating eye contact, are unavailable to the blind
child. If the listener is close by, then initiating
physical contact, for instance, by touching (Example
5) or pinching (Example 6) may be effective, if not
always socially acceptable.

Example 5. Adult₁, Adult₂, SC, and Robert are in
            the classroom. Adult₁ has been talking
            to Adult₂ and SC, not to Robert.
            Robert: [feeling Adult₁'s clothes] *Do
                     you have a dress?*
            Adult₁: *Do I?*
            Robert: *Or pants?*
            Adult₁: *I have on pants.*

Example 6. Robert is sitting next to Denise (SC)
            during group time in kindergarten. He
            pinches her.
            Denise: *Ah!*
            Robert: *What's your name?*
            Denise: *You pincheded* [sic] *me.*
            Robert: *What's your name?*
            Denise: *Denise*

Making some kind of non-linguistic noise may also be
successful (Example 7).

Example 7. Adult₁ has been talking to Joshua, then
            leaves. Adult₂ is nearby.
            Joshua: [making some grunting noises]

Example 7.   Adult₂: *What a silly noise that was.*
(cont'd)   Joshua: [makes more noises]
              Adult₂: *Hey, what kind of noise is*
                       that?

Consider also the attention-attracting 'fake' cough
that Rowland noted in one of her pre-verbal subjects
(1980, p. 95).
     Although using non-verbal devices is one avail-
able option, these five-year old blind children relied most heavily on verbal means to elicit listener
attention, sometimes in conjunction with physical
contact, as in Examples 5 and 6, but often alone.
These verbal devices included vocatives (Example 8),
expressive particles (Example 9), greeting terms
(Example 10) and questions (Example 11).

Example 8.   Alex, Adult₁ and Adult₂ are sitting to-
              gether at a picnic table.
              Alex   : *Mom? I mean...I mean-um...I*
                        mean-um...um...Laura? [=Adult₁]
              Adult₁: *Yeah?*
              Alex   : *I mean, Randa?* [=Adult₂]
              Adult₂: *Yeah? What?* [pause] *Yes,*
                        what do you want?

Example 9.   Alex is playing with the power controls
              on the car seat. Adult₁ and Adult₂ are
              seated nearby.
              Alex   : *Whoops.* [seat is stuck]
              Adult₁: *Whoops, what?* [goes to inves-
                        tigate]

Example 10.   Robert and Adult₁ are in the kindergar-
              ten classroom. Adult₂ enters.
              Adult₁: *Who came in the classroom right*
                        now?
              Robert: *Donny. Hi, Donny.* [=Adult₂]
              Adult₂: *Hello.*

Example 11.   Alex, Adult₁ and Adult₂ are talking
              about piñatas. Then Adult₁ directs some
              commands to Adult₂.
              Alex   : [interrupting] *Are piñatas*
                        heavy to carry?
              Adult₂: *I guess it depends on how big*
                        they are.

Vocatives and questions are especially effective in
eliciting a verbal response from the listener, a
clear sign that he is paying attention. They were

very frequently used by the children in my study,
such that up to one third of all their utterances in
some samples were questions. Urwin also reports the
early and persistent use of such devices for eliciting listener response in at least one of her subjects, Suzanne, who began using the expression *Ay?*
by the age of twelve months (1978, pp. 341-9).

Assessing the Listener's Attention to Referent X

The blind children's difficulties here will be similar to those of assessing the listener's attention
to the speaker, at least in situations where the
referent is found in the physical surroundings.
Again, they miss all visual cues as to the focus of
listener attention, such as direction of gaze, so
they may misjudge it (Examples 12-13).

Example 12.   Robert and Adult$_1$ are walking through
              the parking lot. Robert hears a motor
              running. There is also a car driving
              away nearby.
              Robert: *I wanna see that car...I wanna
                        say hi.*
              Adult$_1$:   [attending to car driving off]
                        Well, that car already left.
              Robert: *No, that car when it's run-
                        ning.*
              Adult$_1$:   *That's a truck.*

Example 13.   Adult$_1$ is helping Robert with an art
              project. Adult$_1$ is gluing tooth-picks
              on the paper; Robert is feeling the tip
              of the metal core of a pipe-cleaner.
              Adult$_1$:   *We're gonna make our ladder
                        nice an' wide.*
              Robert: *Is it pi- is it got a pin in
                        it?*
              Adult$_1$:   *What?*
              Robert: *Put a pin in.*
              Adult$_1$:   *A pin?*

The blind child's problem is compounded, of course,
because he may not perceive all aspects of the
situation which could attract, or distract, the attention of a sighted listener. Thus in Example 12,
Robert seems initially unaware that there is a second vehicle that the adult could be paying attention
to.
      In contexts where the referent is not physical-
ly available, blind children are in basically the

same position as the sighted. They must determine
whether the intended referent 'exists' in the ongoing discourse, that is, whether it is already on the
listener's mind. Or the referent entity may potentially 'exist' in the shared knowledge of the speaker and listener; again the child must judge whether
a particular listener is likely to have access to
the same past experiences or the same knowledge of
the broader context as he does. Being able to see
bestows no particular advantages when it comes to
assessing whether the listener is attending to the
same piece of the invisible world as the speaker.
The kinds of misassessments that blind children make
are very like those of sighted children (Example
14).

Example 14. Alex, Adult1, and Adult2 are talking
             together. Neither Adult1 nor Adult2
             was present when Alex had his 'Big
             Bounce' (a kind of toy).
             Alex   : *You remember when I had a Big*
                       Bounce?
             Adult1: *A Big Bounce?*
             Alex   : *Yeah.*
             Adult2: *(Where) was that?*
             Adult1: *I don't remember that. Was I*
                       there?
             Alex   : *What?*
             Adult1: *I don't think I was there when*
                       you had a Big Bounce.
             Alex   : *Oh.*

Directing Listener Attention to Referent X

Again the blind child's range of options for directing a listener's attention to a physical referent is
more limited than the sighted child's. He cannot
just look at X, indicating his focus of attention by
his direction of gaze. Nor do blind children point
to objects that attract their attention or spontaneously show objects to others. For the most part,
they are limited in their non-verbal attention-
directing strategies to physical contact with the
referent, like touching (Example 15) or holding (Example 16). Sometimes they may try to bring the listener into contact with the focal object as well
(Example 17).

Example 15. Alex and Adult1 are sitting in the car.
             Alex: [touching the button on the car
                    door that controls the window]

Example 15.   Alex: *Is that the window shade opener?*
(cont'd)

Example 16.   Alex, Adult$_1$ and Adult$_2$ are sitting in
the car. Alex is holding a bag of can-
dies.
Alex: *This is a candy bag that -*
that - an' it has candy.

Example 17.   Robert and Joshua are sitting at a
small table. Joshua is practising on
the Braille writer, which Robert would
like to use. Robert pushes a spiral
notebook at Joshua, getting it in his
way.
Robert: *Here's your notebook, Josh.*
Joshua: *No.*
Robert: *Here's you- here's your note-*
book, Joshua.
Joshua: *No!*
Robert: *You-(right) here's your note-*
book.

Blind children are much less constrained by their
impairment, however, once they begin to use verbal
attention-directing strategies. They can name or
describe what they are attending to, either alone,
as in Examples 18 and 19, or in conjunction with a
non-verbal strategy, as in Example 17 above.

Example 18.   Alex, Adult$_1$, and Adult$_2$ are walking
through the park and pass close to the
corral by the pony ride.
Alex :   *I smell the ponies!* [adults
laugh]
Adult$_1$: *So do I. They stink.*

Example 19.   In the car. Alex had been playing with
the motorized control to raise and
lower the driver's seat. Now he is
sitting on the passenger side. Adult$_1$
runs the motor to adjust the seat.
Alex :   [teasing voice] *Who's making*
that seat go up an' down?
Adult$_1$: *I'm makin' it go forward so I*
can reach the pedals.

Referring to X with a Definite, Unambiguous Referring Expression

Several recent studies of blind children's semantic development (Herron, 1974; Bernstein, 1980; Mulford, 1981; Landau, Chapter 7), as well as the earlier discussions of "verbalism" (e.g. Cutsforth, 1932; Nolan, 1960; Harley, 1963; Dokecki, 1966), have focussed on the issue of blind children learning to use referring expressions accurately. Blind children, like sighted ones, have to learn how to use language to pick out precisely and uniquely the entity or entities they are focussing on. Both must learn the definiteness conditions on referring expressions. Although all children typically have problems in learning to use some kinds of words correctly, the blind child may face additional difficulties with words whose referents are primarily or partially distinguished by visually-perceived attributes. The most obvious examples of problem domains are totally visual words like colour terms or *light-dark* (see Millar, Chapter 15). Other classes of words may also pose problems because the information necessary to correctly identify and label the categories they refer to is most readily perceived visually. For example, two of the children reported on here had difficulty for a time with the pronouns *he* and *she*, so that they sometimes used *he* for girls and *she* for boys. The interesting point was that these confusions only occurred when they were talking about other children, not about adults. It is not hard to imagine that the clues sighted speakers generally use to distinguish five-year old boys from five-year old girls are relatively unavailable to a blind child and that the clues he must rely on, such as voice, relative size or even clothing, are not always sufficient for identification. Example 12 above is also a case where the child makes a perceptual misidentification, calling a truck a car based on its sound, and thus confusing the listener temporarily. Further problems arise, too, because blind children may not always be aware of potential referential ambiguities in the speech context, as in Example 20.

Example 20.   Joshua is feeling a ring on Adult's hand; there are two rings there.
Joshua: *I want the ring on.*
Adult :   *Which-which ring?*
Joshua: *I (wanna) put the ring on.*
Adult :   *Which ring?*
Joshua: *I put the ring on.*

Example 20. Adult : *Which ring? My little ring?*
(cont'd)   Joshua: *Yeah.*
             Adult : *Or my big ring?*
             Joshua: *My* [sic] *little ring. Big
                      ring.*
             Adult : *My big ring. O.K.*

Joshua does not seem to have noticed that there are
two rings and that therefore the phrase *the ring* is
not definite enough. Particular kinds of expressions (e.g. spatial deictics) may take a very long
time for blind children to learn to use with complete referential accuracy. Some words may never be
used with just the same meanings by blind and sighted speakers.[2]

DISCUSSION

Although a number of examples have been presented
here to illustrate various kinds of referential
problems faced by blind speakers, it should be
pointed out that, generally speaking, these three
five-year olds were quite successful referrers, at
least judging by the responses of their listeners.
Two main factors seem to account for their relative
referential success.
     First, by the age of five, these blind children
have already mastered a number of effective verbal
and non-verbal devices for establishing reference.
They have become relatively proficient at assessing
listener attention and, if anything, may err in the
direction of 'over-attracting' attention by an ex-
cessive use of vocatives and questions. Although
they are still learning the conventional uses of
some kinds of referring expressions, they make few
blatant meaning errors. We need more detailed information on the use of referential devices by
sighted children of the same age in similar settings
for comparison, of course, but one suspects that the
performance of the two groups will be similar.
     The second factor which contributes to these
children's apparent referential success is the very
active role of their adult listeners as interpreters
of intended reference. In all these speech samples,
the children were interacting with familiar and attentive adults, for the most part in surroundings
also very familiar to the child. The adults were
able to exploit their knowledge of the particular
children and, in almost all cases, arrived at interpretations of potentially ambiguous utterances which

seemed to correspond to the children's intentions. Of course, all conversations involve listener inter- pretation as well as speaker intention, and the par- ents of sighted children as well as blind ones typi- cally need to read a lot into their youngster's ear- ly communicative attempts. It seems clear, however, that successful interaction with blind children re- quires some special skills in assessing their foci of attention and in interpreting their utterances from the perspective of a speaker without vision. As Fraiberg (1977) and Rowland (1980) have suggest- ed, some of these skills may have to be taught to people who have not had experience with blind chil- dren. It is also a common practice to teach blind children some of the gestural conventions for indi- cating attention, for example, turning to face the person one is addressing. This type of training may facilitate their communication with unfamiliar lis- teners to some extent. It is necessary to gather more data on how referentially successful blind speakers are, both children and adults, in situa- tions where their listeners are relatively unfamil- iar and unskilled interpreters.

Much more information is also needed on the de- velopment of referential skills among younger blind children. Although Rowland (1980) and Urwin (1978a) have made valuable contributions with their studies of children under the age of three, there are still many unanswered questions. We can anticipate that problems of referring will be especially severe for the younger language-learning blind child for two reasons. First, the young sighted child talks pri- marily about his immediate surroundings and relies heavily on non-verbal means for assessing, attract- ing and directing attention. Many, if not most, of these strategies involve vision. Not only is the blind child's perception of his physical surround- ings more limited than the sighted child's, but he also lacks access to those non-verbal attentional strategies that depend on vision. Secondly, al- though blind children may eventually learn to use verbal devices very successfully to accomplish ref- erence, the development of a repertoire of such strategies is undoubtedly gradual. What is more, among sighted children, the use of certain verbal devices is normally preceded by the use of conven- tional non-verbal devices. For instance, sighted children only begin to use pointing words like *that* or *there* after they have come to use pointing ges- tures; the words first appear only in combination with the gestures (Bates, 1976; E. Clark, 1978).

Since young blind children do not use these conventional gestures, language acquisition data from blind children should help to resolve the issue of whether such gestures are in fact prerequisites for specific, verbal developments or only typical precursors. The answer which seems to be emerging from Rowland and Urwin's work is that blind children can master the verbal devices without first having recourse to the non-**verbal** ones, but that their development proceeds along a somewhat different course, possibly through the use of unconventional gestures and/or language rituals, and perhaps at a different pace than that of sighted children.

CONCLUSION

This discussion of referential development in blind children has been intended to outline in some detail the range of problems which need to be investigated. Only very sketchy solutions to these problems exist so far. This paper has concentrated only on the development of the blind child as a speaker, but certainly his complementary role as listener and interpreter of reference needs to be explored, too, to arrive at a broader understanding of how he learns to communicate. As more is learned about how and to what extent individual blind children overcome the potential obstacles their impairment poses, child language researchers will be in a better position to suggest ways of enhancing the development of referential communication among young blind speakers. Ultimately, we should have a better understanding of the necessary, as opposed to the characteristic, role of vision in the development of the referential function of language.

NOTES

1. This chapter is based on portions of my unpublished doctoral dissertation "Talking without Seeing: Some Problems of Semantic Development in Blind Children", Stanford University, 1981.
2. I will skirt entirely the issue of whether or not any two speakers, sighted or blind, ever use the same word with precisely the same meaning.

Chapter 10.

EFFECTANCE MOTIVATION AND THE DEVELOPMENT OF COMMU-
NICATIVE COMPETENCE IN BLIND AND SIGHTED CHILDREN

Harry McGurk

A number of issues recur in the chapters of this
volume, three of which I wish to select for particular discussion. These are issues, it seems to me,
which must be resolved if we are ever to make progress in this area. Firstly, I wish to consider the
nature of the samples involved in research on the
development of communication in blind children,
secondly, to consider the extent to which there are
specific factors in the development of communicative
competence which are attributable to the absence of
visual input, and thirdly, the extent to which there
may be differences between totally blind and partially-sighted children in their acquisition of communicative competence. Throughout this discussion
my perspective will be that of a developmental psychologist rather than that of a linguist, and I will
illustrate my comments with reference to psychological research.

SAMPLE HETEROGENEITY IN RESEARCH ON COMMUNICATIVE
COMPETENCE IN BLIND CHILDREN

It has been repeatedly pointed out, for example by
Elstner (Chapter 3) and Schaner-Wolles (Chapter 4),
that visually-impaired children are frequently handicapped in other ways in addition to their deficient
visual experience. These additional handicaps tend
to confound the interpretation of data when it comes
to assessing the extent to which any communicative
delay or deviance shown by such children may be attributed directly to their visual deficit. One solution to this problem is to conduct research with
subjects whose sole handicap is visual, as reported,
for example, by Barbara Landau (Chapter 7). Moreover, if it is possible to select subjects whose

handicap varies in degree from total blindness,
through a moderate degree of visual impairment to
normal vision, then we can assess the extent to
which dependent variables are also transitively ordered between subjects from the different categories. If such transitive ordering is observed, then
we can be confident that the phenomena under scrutiny are related to blindness.

However, such a strategy raises other, equally
important methodological and ethical questions. The
population to which the results of a study designed
along the above lines could be generalized is clearly a minority one among visually-handicapped children; as we have noted above, the vast majority of
such children are also handicapped in other ways.
We also noted above, however, that only by working
with otherwise normal children who happen to be visually-handicapped can we learn what, if anything, is
specifically visual about the development of communicative competence. In this sense, we are using
the occurrence of the congenital visual defect as a
natural experiment, a context in which to evaluate
hypotheses about the role of vision in the development of communication. Perhaps in so doing we need
to acknowledge explicitly that it is the blind who
are serving us and our theories, rather than we who
are serving the blind. Of course, data from research designed to address theoretical issues can
serve as a basis for the development of strategies
to enhance the acquisition of communicative skills
among children from handicapped populations. However, the development of such strategies needs also
to be addressed directly and it is a moot point
whether the interests of the modal visually-handicapped child are served by research investigations
on samples from highly restricted populations.

DOES VISUAL HANDICAP HAVE SPECIFIC EFFECTS ON THE
DEVELOPMENT OF COMMUNICATIVE COMPETENCE?

In Chapter 2, Wode raised the question of whether
the visually-impaired, but otherwise normal, child
showed deviant patterns of communication, or whether
such children were merely delayed in arriving at
communicative competence. The question can also be
asked whether, should deviance indeed be manifested,
it can be causally attributed to lack of, or reduced, visual input *per se*, or whether there are
other factors which covary with visual handicap but
which contributed more directly to the development

of communication. The bulk of the evidence presented in the other chapters of this volume suggests
that blindness is associated with delayed rather
than deviant communicative development. Only the
data presented by Anne Mills (Chapter 5) and by
Barbara Dodd (Chapter 6) have revealed highly specific effects attributable to blindness and these
were confined to a fairly circumscribed, though
theoretically significant, aspect of phonological
development. In the main, the evidence reported
here indicates that, although he takes longer to
traverse the route, the visually-impaired child follows the same path to communicative competence as
his sighted peers, and the level of competence he
eventually achieves is well within the range of reaction we accept as normality. Visual impairment,
rather than having specific, determinate effects,
thus seems to have general moderating or modulating
influences upon the development of communicative
competence.

R.W. White (1959) has argued that there is an
endogenous, overarching human psychological motive
to be effective, to have reliable effects, to be
competent in exchanges with the physical and social
environment. This effectance motivation is enhanced
by experiences of agency, of events in the world being contingent upon one's behaviour. On such experience is the motivation to acquire competence
based. With respect to the development of communicative competence work by Kaye (1977) and Collis and
Schaffer (1975) suggest how normal patterns of care-
taker-child interaction serve to provide the infant
and young child with the experience of such contingency within the context of communicative exchanges.
Kaye's analysis of feeding episodes shows how mothers of newborn babies monitor the infant's sucking
rhythms and interpolate such behaviour as talking to
the baby or adjusting body posture into the pauses
between sucking bursts. These interpolations have
the effect of lengthening such filled pauses relative to unfilled pauses. Thus, the on-off pattern
of infant sucking influences the phasing of maternal
caretaking behaviour and this, in turn, influences
the temporal relationship between pausing and sucking. Kaye argues that the origins of dialogue are
to be found in these reciprocally contingent, turn-
taking exchanges between infant and mother.

Collis and Schaffer (1975), working with
twelve-month old infants and their mothers, illustrate how the mother, by monitoring the direction of
infant regard, identifies the focus of infant atten-

tion and may comment appropriately. Thus, the infant's visual behaviour specifies a topic upon which the mother provides commentary. Murphy and Messer (1977) also show how direction of regard, pointing and other deictic behaviour on the part of the normal infant provide opportunities for contingent exchange between infant and caretaker.

The absence of such visually mediated deictic behaviours from the repertoire of the blind or visually-impaired child severely constrains the opportunities for contingent interaction over shared referents both before and during language acquisition. Very young sighted infants produce their own visual and other referential gestures and can follow the gestural referents of others. The visually-impaired child thus misses out on a whole range of opportunities for self and other initiated contingent exchanges and, to that extent his competence-enhancing experiences are restricted. Such restrictions can be expected to have a generalized delay effect upon language acquisition.

Some of the filmed material presented during this conference, together with comments made by Edna Adelson in her paper (Chapter 1), confirm that visually-impaired children do display components of the orienting reaction other than direction of visual regard. For example, on introduction of new or novel objects or events they show interruption of ongoing behaviour and general stilling. A sensitive adult can use such behaviours as a guide for specifying topics on which to comment and thereby enhance the contingency experience of the child. In so doing, the adult enhances his or her own contingency in interaction with the child; from the film material and from observations by Adelson it is evident that contingencies are deficient for <u>both</u> adult and child in interaction sequences involving blind children. Thus, the blind child may not only have a reduced sense of agency, but is also deficient in providing contingent feedback in interaction with others. Unless steps are taken to overcome this deficiency, it can only serve further to reduce the child's contingency related experience and to delay further the development of communicative competence.

Because the blind child's non-verbal behaviour so often fails to provide topics for comment, parents frequently adopt an interrogative mode in interaction with blind children. Moreover, data attest to the fact that parents of blind children employ direct questions to the child with much greater frequency than do parents of sighted children.

Although questioning may facilitate a rudimentary form of turn-taking between parent and child, because the initiative is always with the interrogator, the practice does not enhance the child's experience of agency. This is particularly so with closed as opposed to open-ended questions. Interestingly, in this regard, some recent work by Blank (1981) has shown that parents of sighted but linguistically retarded children employ many more questions during parent-child interaction sequences compared with parents whose children display normal language development. Of course, there is something of a chicken and egg problem here, but Blank's work also suggests that the adoption of a freer interactive style with language-delayed children does enhance the quality of their linguistic output. It might be valuable to determine whether the same holds true with respect to the development of communicative competence in blind children, for here also we have a factor which may be implicated in the general deficiency in these children's linguistic development.

COMMUNICATIVE COMPETENCE IN BLIND COMPARED WITH PARTIALLY-SIGHTED CHILDREN

In this area there is a considerable amount of potentially conflicting evidence. For example, in Walter Elstner's study (Chapter 3) he observed that the partially-sighted subjects showed the same degree of speech and language impairment as the totally blind. As we noted previously, however, Elstner's sample was a very heterogeneous one and the probability exists that additional handicaps contributed to linguistic impairment of the blind and partially-sighted alike. On the other hand, Barbara Landau (Chapter 7) stressed that in her work with otherwise normal children little difference was revealed between the language performance of blind, partially-sighted and normal children with respect to such general measures as mean length of utterance (MLU). During discussion at this conference, cases were reported which were at variance with these observations, cases involving substantial differences in communicative competence between blind and partially-sighted subjects, the latter being much closer to the normally sighted than the former.

It seems important, for theoretical and for practical reasons, that this issue should be addressed and resolved. Resolution, of course, will

require careful description of the degree of visual
impairment manifested by partially-sighted subjects
and its relationship to communicative competence
across a range of linguistic and paralinguistic variables. The pay-off for such detailed analysis is
potentially considerable. At a theoretical level,
the outcome would enhance our understanding of those
specifically visual processes which may contribute
to the development of communicative competence.
Practically, such work would be of importance for
the development of intervention procedures directed
towards maximizing the potential utilization of
residual vision in the developing child. Irene
Neilson (1981) has illustrated how spatial cognition
and spatial mobility can be facilitated by intervention programmes initiated early in the partially-
sighted child's infancy; if intervention is delayed,
then little benefit accrues thereby. With this in
mind we would do well to inform ourselves whether
partial vision is of significance to the acquisition
of communicative competence, and, if so, to determine whether its effectiveness can be enhanced by
specifically developed, appropriately timed, intervention strategies. In such fashion it may be possible to work toward attaining for the partially-
sighted in the field of communicative competence
what Neilson has been attaining for them in the
field of spatial mobility. Were we to begin to realize such aspirations then we would have begun to
serve the blind and partially-sighted child. Otherwise we are in danger of continuing to need the
blind more than they need us.

Chapter 11.

PATTERNS OF INTERACTION BETWEEN THREE BLIND INFANTS
AND THEIR MOTHERS

Charity Rowland

INTRODUCTION

The early communicative ability of visually-impaired
children has received little attention until recently, probably because visual impairment *per se* has
not been regarded as an impediment to the eventual
acquisition of language skills. Although speech
problems are more prevalent among blind than sighted
children (Miner, 1963; Graham, 1966; Elstner, Chapter 3), the linguistic ability of the average blind
child without concomitant handicaps has been reported on a par with the sighted child of the same age
(Fraiberg, 1977). Burlingham (1961) found that an
initial delay in vocabulary acquisition had been
surmounted by school age, and found no deficit in
syntactic abilities among blind children.
     The lack of language problems associated with
visual deficits is surprising, given that the blind
infant typically displays significant delays in
gross motor development, cognitive development and
psycho-social development. It is only recently that
attention has been focused on the early stages of
language development, including the pre-verbal abilities of blind children.
     Fraiberg (1977) described the average blind in-
fant as communicatively rather unresponsive, with a
restricted range of facial expressions and a suspected low rate of spontaneous vocalizations. She
described the pre-verbal communication system of the
blind infant as a system of "smile" and "hand" language that substitutes for the "eye" language of the
sighted infant. The reported research investigated
such suspected behavioural differences between blind
and sighted infants through the micro-analysis of
communicative behaviours of pre-verbal blind children and their mothers.

114

The study was guided by convergent trends in the recent literatures in language acquisition and developmental psychology. The first trend derives from an abundance of developmental research (Lewis and Rosenblum, 1977; Schaffer, 1977), that describes the extremely sophisticated receptive and signalling abilities of the human neonate that are evident in vocal and visual exchanges. The second trend derives from the revival of interest in a pragmatic approach to language development - one which ascribes the functional properties of language to certain pre-verbal behaviours (Dore, 1974, 1975; Halliday, 1979). A request, for instance, may be realized before the acquisition of formal language, through non-verbal behaviours such as pointing, visual regard or fussing. Early play activities and turn-taking rituals especially are considered important precursors to formal language (Bruner, 1974/5). In the words of R. Clark (1978, p. 234), language is considered a "progressive complication of the basic communicative function".

In a longitudinal, correlational study with empirical implications for this approach, Bates et al. (1977) found several good predictors of language development in the pre-verbal abilities of sighted children aged 9-13 months. These predictors included conventional gestures, such as pointing and showing, symbolic and combinatorial play, imitation and tool use. The authors interpreted their data as support for a common substrate for both pre-linguistic communication and language - a substrate that may be described as a capacity for communication through the use of conventional signs. Such studies as this formed the theoretical perspective that guided the behavioural observations of this study.

The four main research questions addressed by the study were:

1. What are the potentially communicative behaviours produced by blind infants and their mothers, and at what rates are these individual behaviours produced?

2. To which maternal behaviours do the blind infants seem to be responsive or non-responsive, as evidenced by temporal relationships between maternal and infant behaviours?

3. To which behaviours do the mothers of blind infants seem to be responsive or non-responsive, as evidenced, again, by temporal contingencies between behaviours?

4. Finally, do blind infants appear to adhere to the same course of development in early

communicative skills as Bates et al. (1977) described for the sighted infant?

METHOD

Subjects
The three subjects described here were congenitally
totally blind. All three infants were female and
were enrolled in a pre-school programme at a university affiliated Child Study Center (CSC) in
Oklahoma. The children, Amy, Maria and Tanya were
11, 15 and 16 months of age, respectively, at the
start of the six-month project. Amy and Maria lived
close enough to the Child Study Center to attend
hour-long individual sessions twice a week. Tanya
attended the Center for longer individual sessions
once a month and attended local special education
classes twice a week. The reported research was
conducted independently of these educational programmes, except that the films of the children were
made available to their teachers at the Center. Although none of the subjects suffered from concomitant sensory handicaps, Amy and Tanya were severely
developmentally delayed. The three infants are pro-
filed in Table 11.1. In the brief descriptions below, the various developmental milestones are listed. For the purpose of comparison, these are followed in square brackets by age-equivalents for
sighted children taken from the Callier-Azusa Scale
(Stillman, 1978).
     Amy was eleven months old at initial observa-
tion. She had no useful vision, suffered from generalized hypotonia and was developmentally delayed
in all areas. Amy sat only with support [4 months],
had poor head control, and would hold objects only
passively, and for no more than a few seconds [3
months]. She seemed happy to be left alone, playing
with her hands and babbling. Interestingly, she
demonstrated excellent head-turn and eye-orientation
to auditory cues [5 months]. By 17 months of age,
she was playing with her hands at midline [4
months], and would play independently with toys.
She could sit unsupported in a high chair, tuck her
legs under her and rock in a crawling position [8
months] and move around the floor a little by rolling and scooting [6 months]. Her auditory localization skills were excellent [12 months] and manual
exploratory behaviour was becoming more purposeful
and frequent [8 months].

Table 11.1: Subject Profile

	Amy	Maria	Tanya
Birthdate	12.77	7.77	6.77
Age at Initiation of Project	11 months	15 months	16 months
Family Income	Low-middle	Low	Low
Home	Urban	Urban	Rural
Ordinal Position in Family	2nd of 2	1st of 1 (but 4th of 4 under 21 yrs. in extended family)	3rd of 3
Others in Home	Mother, father, 1 sibling	Mother, 2 aunts, uncle, grandmother, various other relatives move in/out	Mother, 2 siblings
Most Recent Visual Assessment	Responds to bright lights (10 months)	None (10 months)	No visual response (13 months)
Visual Diagnosis	Visual impairment; cortical basis	Congenital anophthalmia	Bilateral optic hypoplasia
Age at Diagnosis of Visual Impairment	6 months	Birth	Prior to 9 months
Concomitant Handicaps	Generalized hypotonia	None	None
Age at First Evaluation by CSC	10 months	3 months	9 months
Vision at Time of Referral to CSC	No consistent response, may see shadows	No visual response	No visual response
Age at Onset of Therapy	11 months	4 months	10 months

She vocalized loudly and fairly frequently; she seemed to understand a few verbal phrases [10 months] and responded to vocal intonation [3 months]. Amy's mother was highly anxious, painstaking in her application of recommended programmes and at the start seemed over-involved with her infant. Her behaviour levels were very high except for vocalization, and she produced a high rate of behaviour combinations. As her child became more independent and competent, however, Amy's mother managed to disengage herself to a certain extent.

Maria was 15 months at initial observation. Born without eyes, her blindness was evident from the start, and educational programming began at four months. Maria was by far the most advanced of the subjects in terms of social, motor and language skills; she was a confident, insatiably sociable baby. At the start of the project, she was trying eagerly to stand up and walk (although she did not crawl) and she would stand unassisted momentarily [10 months]. She imitated some words as well as non-linguistic vocalizations such as coughing and sneezing [12 months]. She could touch several body parts and wave good-bye on command [18 months]. By the end of the project, at the age of 21 months, Maria had taken as many as six steps by herself [11 months] and had been 'cruising' around the house for several months [10 months]. She had a vocabulary of about 20 words which she used in up to three-word combinations [24 months].

Maria's mother was a 16-year old high-school student when her baby was born. She was a warm, effusive girl, who continued to live with her own family after the birth of her child. She did not seem very attentive to professional recommendations, preferring to interact more spontaneously with her daughter. An environmental variable that set this infant apart from the other subjects was the large size of the family. Maria interacted virtually ceaselessly with a relatively large number of people. This family situation, combined with the fact that her handicap was evident at birth, no doubt contributed to her rapid development. When she was four months of age, Maria's mother and her grandmother began receiving training in tactile, vestibular, locomotor and language stimulation for Maria. Some of the training was then passed on to other members of the large extended family. Thus, effective interaction patterns that were appropriate to Maria's sensory abilities were established early on with a relatively large number of partners. (Amy

118

and Tanya, in contrast, were not even diagnosed as visually-impaired until they were six months of age.)

At 16 months, Tanya was developmentally delayed in all areas and showed no visual response. She was a passive, contented baby who was able to sit unassisted [7 months] and had once sat herself up [8 months]. Once in sitting position, however, she tended to engage in self-stimulatory behaviour. She could push herself up into a crawling position and let herself down, and her tactile exploration was proceeding well. By the end of the project (at 22 months), Tanya had begun to move around the house by rolling [6 months]. She could sit herself up, lie back down, and rock back and forth in a crawling position [8 months]. She explored faces very carefully with her hands, and searched well in any direction both to a sound cue [12 months] and in quest of temporarily abandoned noiseless toys [9 months]. Her range of vocalizations had increased, and she had begun to say *mama*, but only imitatively [12 months]. At the start of the project, Tanya's mother was quite restrained in vocalization and touching behaviour. Her interactions with Tanya tended to focus on inanimate objects and her general behaviour level was low. By the end of the project, she had become much warmer and more engaged. Her touching and vocal behaviour had increased, while her production of noise using inanimate objects had decreased.

Procedures and Analysis

Films of mother-infant interactions were made in the subjects' homes at regular intervals over a six-month period to document the development of communicative skills within each dyad. Mothers were instructed to play with their children in as natural a manner as possible during filming. Approximately one-half of the filmed sessions were structured by the introduction of a standard set of toys not available in the subjects' home. The remaining sessions did not involve inanimate objects. The films were analyzed at two-second intervals for seven categories of infant behaviour and three categories of maternal behaviour, comprising a total of 42 subcategories. The coding system is described below.

Code Development

The observational coding system was developed from a combination of theory, intuition and practice on the

preliminary data. The code was revised frequently
to accomodate the first sets of filmed data as they
became available for analysis. The rationale for
the code developed from the following considerations:

1. The communicative behaviours of mother and
infant were of primary interest.

2. From the perspective of the blind infant,
many of the potentially communicative behaviours of
the mother (such as facial expression and visual regard) are functionally non-existent. Therefore, the
scoring of maternal behaviours was limited to those
observable behaviours that could be sensed by a
sightless infant. (No doubt the infants also responded to certain other maternal stimuli such as
breath, body temperature and odour - but since these
variables were neither observable nor subject to the
mothers' voluntary control, they were not coded.)

3. From the maternal point of view, however,
almost any infant behaviour might be considered expressive, so that almost all categories of gross infant behaviour were coded.

4. Initially it had been hoped that both verbal and non-verbal infant behaviours would be cod-
able. When only one infant demonstrated any verbal
behaviour, special attention was paid to the presence of the conventional pre-verbal gestures. However, the number of conventional gestures was also
so low, that it quickly became obvious that a more
molecular level of analysis was required than had
originally been anticipated. Thus, attention came
to be focussed upon more idiosyncratic expressive
activities of the infants.

The coded behaviour categories appear in Table
11.2. A minimum of 80 per cent inter-observer
agreement was achieved between two observers for
each behaviour category for each subject. Data were
first analyzed for the frequency of behaviours.
Many subcategories (the majority) did not occur sufficiently frequently to warrant further analysis.
Where subcategories could be meaningfully collapsed
into larger categories, this was done (for instance,
linguistic and non-linguistic vocalizations were
collapsed). Where collapsing subcategories was not
feasible, the low-frequency behaviour categories
were excluded from further analysis.

Table 11.2: List of Coded Behaviours

Infant

A. Non-vocal Sound
B. Vocal Sound
    1. linguistic
    2. non-linguistic
    3. imitation of maternal vocalization
C. Head Gestures
D. Facial Expression
    1. positive
    2. negative
E. Manual Activity
    1. spontaneous gesture
    2. elicited gesture
    3. exploration of space
    4. reach for mother
    5. reach for object
    6. release mother
    7. release object
    8. explore mother
    9. explore object
    10. manipulate mother
    11. manipulate object
    12. hold mother
    13. hold object
    14. withdraw hand from mother
    15. withdraw hand from object
    16. push away mother
    17. push away object
    18. touch self
F. Whole Body Movement
    1. approach
    2. avoidance
G. Stereotypic Behaviour
    1. with object
    2. with self
    3. self-abusive

Mother

H. Tactile Behaviour
    1. caress
    2. restrain
    3. direct
I. Vocal Sound
    1. linguistic
    2. non-linguistic
J. Non-vocal Sound

RESULTS

Communicative Repertoires of the Infants

Frequency data for the individual behaviour categories of mothers and infants have been described in
an earlier paper (Rowland, 1981). Table 11.3 presents the proportion of scored intervals containing
a few selected behaviours for each pair of subjects.
Highlights of these data follow.[1]

Table 11.3: Comparison of Pairs on Occurrence of Selected Behaviours: Proportion of Intervals Containing Each Behaviour

	Infant Behaviours	Amy	Maria	Tanya
b A	Non-vocal Sound[a]	.17	.26	.25
B 1,2,3	Vocalization	.29	.23	.19
D 1	Positive Facial Expression	.08	.23	.30
D 2	Negative Facial Expression	.07	.03	.00
E 1	Spontaneous Manual Gesture	.01	.06	.09
E 3	Explore Space	.03	.17	.00
E 11	Manipulate Object[a]	.19	.31	.27
E 9	Explore Object[a]	.06	.04	.10
E 8	Explore Mother	.00	.02	.05
E 5	Reach for Object[a]	.01	.20	.17
E 18	Touch Self	.35	.03	.10
	No Manual Activity	.46	.24	.33
	Maternal Behaviours	Amy	Maria	Tanya
H 1,2,3	Touch	.87	.53	.67
I 1,2	Vocalization	.44	.66	.56
J	Non-vocal Sound[a]	.56	.24	.30
	Vocal Imitation of Infant	.01	.03	.00

Note: a. Proportions generated from toy sequences only.
Note: b. Numbering system references the equivalent coded
behaviours from Table 11.2.

Infant vocalizations occurred in at least 19
per cent of all intervals across subjects. Significantly, none of the mothers considered their infants
to be particularly quiet, and all mothers reported
high rates of vocalization by their infants when

they were left alone. Only Maria, however, who was by far the most advanced in all developmental areas, produced any linguistic vocalizations. Facial expressions (positive and negative combined) occurred in at least 15 per cent of intervals across subjects. Independent manual activity, which had been expected to be relatively frequent, was completely absent in at least 24 per cent of intervals across subjects (see Table 11.3; Item: No Manual Activity). Spontaneous manual gestures, which included idiosyncratic movements of hands or arms, occurred in an average of 5 per cent of intervals across subjects. Examples of these gestures appear in Table 11.4. No conventional gestures such as giving or reaching as a request were observed in the infants.

The mothers exhibited high rates of touching, which were undoubtedly related to the postural maturity of their respective infants. Amy's mother touched her daughter, who was unable to sit unsupported, almost 100 per cent of the time. Maria's mother touched her daughter, who had good locomotor skills, least frequently (about 50 per cent of the time).

Table 11.4: Examples of Spontaneous Manual Gestures

Subject	Age (months)	Examples
Amy	11	Fingers on left hand play – hand moves slightly as mother squeezes ball at her
	11	Right hand, with index finger extended, waivers as she cries
	14	Pats stomach
	17	Throws arms and head back, starting to vocalize in protest
Maria	15	Right arm darts out suddenly as she laughs
	16	Waves and claps hands excitedly
	16	Lifts hands to face
Tanya	16	Brings arms up as mother shakes slinky toy
	17	Arms go up, hands go to head, brush head, arms go down, but stay extended (as she smiles)
	18	Bats arms, claps hands

The mother's vocalization rates were also high (occurring in at least 44 per cent of scored intervals), but the mothers rarely imitated their infants' vocalizations. Significantly, Maria's mother
was most likely to imitate her infant's vocalizations, which were frequently linguistic.

Directions of Effects

Following the frequency analyses, the sequences of
behaviours for each subject pair were analyzed for
interdependencies over time using a lagged condition-
al probabilities programme developed by G. Sackett
(1979, 1980). This nonparametric technique compares
the observed (or contingent) probability of a target
behaviour, given the antecedent occurrence of a criterion behaviour at any specified time lag, with its
expected (or chance) probability of occurrence over
an entire series of sequential observations.

This 'lag' technique is extremely costly and
easily produces unmanageable amounts of data. Furthermore, 'fishing expeditions' into the dependen-
cies between large numbers of behaviours produced by
interacting individuals are bound to yield numerous
chance relationships. Therefore, the 'lag' analyses
were used only to investigate pairs of behaviours
that were expected to be highly temporally related,
either by virtue of the theoretical assumptions of
the research, or as a result of actual observations
of the mother-infant interactions. Thus, a very
limited set of behavioural contingencies was examined. In this paper, discussion will centre around
the analysis of temporal relationships between Infant Smiles, Gestures, and Vocalizations and Maternal Touch and Vocalizations (see Table 11.3).

In the sighted mother-infant pair, behavioural
reciprocity, or mutual responsivity, is observed at
a very early age. Condon and Sander (1974) found
that "micro-kinesic" behaviours of neonates were responsive to maternal speech; Tronick, Als and
Brazelton (1975) found a conversational quality in
the vocal exchanges of three-month old infants and
their mothers; Stern, Jaffe, Beebe and Bennett
(1975) discuss mutual reciprocity in the visual and
vocal exchanges of mothers and infants. Although we
cannot concisely quantify or compare the degree of
behavioural reciprocity displayed by the mother-infant dyads of this study, it is clear that the infants affected their mothers' behaviour much more
strongly and systematically than the mothers affected the infant's behaviour. When we examine the

probabilities of specific infant behaviours following specific maternal behaviours at the immediately
succeeding interval, we see a striking lack of responsiveness of infant behaviour. A similar analysis of the probabilities of maternal behaviours following specific infant behaviours at the immediately
succeeding interval revealed that mothers responded
rapidly and frequently to infant behaviours and particularly to Infant Smile. In order to test the
consistency of these immediate or lag-1 effects, two
statistics, called the Magnitude and Z_{sum} were computed for each subject pair across the first ten intervals (20 seconds) following a given behaviour.
Magnitude describes the extent to which contingent
probabilities exceed chance in either direction, av-
eraged over a specified number of lags. The larger
the Magnitude, the more predictable is the change in
the frequency of the contingent event, given a specified antecedent event. The Z_{sum} describes general
trends in the direction of change: a large positive
Z_{sum} implies a reliable excitation of the contingent
behaviour, while a negative Z_{sum} implies an inhibition of the contingent behaviour. The computed statistics for these temporal relationships appear in
Table 11.5.

The upper half of Table 11.5 displays statistics for the contingent probabilities of Maternal
Touch and Maternal Vocalization following three different infant behaviours (Vocalization, Gesture and
Smile). For each subject pair, the Magnitude of
Maternal Vocalization was highest following Infant
Smile. The Z_{sums} for Maternal Touch and Vocalization following Infant Smile are uniformly positive
and significant ($p < .001$), indicating a reliable
excitation of maternal behaviours in response to Infant Smile. For Amy and Tanya, the maternal response following Infant Vocalization was of very low
Magnitude with non-significant Z_{sums}. For Maria,
however, the Magnitudes of maternal behaviours following Infant Vocalizations were higher, and the
Z_{sums} positive and significant ($p < .001$). The
sharp contrast in maternal response following
Maria's vocalizations may reflect the fact that many
of her vocalizations were actual words, while the
other infants produced only non-linguistic vocalizations. Interestingly, the mothers of Amy and Tanya,
who did not have infant words to respond to, did appear to be more responsive than Maria's mother to
Infant Gestures, as evidenced by the significant
Z_{sums} associated with Maternal Touch and Vocalization following Infant Gestures.

125

Table 11.5: Magnitude and Zsums of Crosslagged Functions[a]

Criterion Behaviour --> Target Behaviour	AMY Magnitude[b]	AMY Zsum[c]	MARIA Magnitude	MARIA Zsum	TANYA Magnitude	TANYA Zsum
Infant Vocalize --> Mother Vocalize	.53	+1.24	1.84	+5.23***	.83	+1.89
Infant Vocalize --> Mother Touch	.66	+1.84	2.69	+7.65***	.49	- .11
Infant Gesture --> Mother Vocalize	2.29	-6.52***	1.17	+2.27	1.56	+4.44**
Infant Gesture --> Mother Touch	1.04	+2.63**	.78	+1.31	1.21	+3.45***
Infant Smile --> Mother Vocalize	2.92	+8.31***	3.14	+6.88***	2.76	+7.86***
Infant Smile --> Mother Touch	1.40	+3.99***	3.80	+10.82***	2.67	+7.60***
Mother Vocalize --> Infant Vocalize	.65	-1.08	.53	+ .71	.75	+1.10
Mother Vocalize --> Infant Gesture	.88	-1.72	.98	+2.76**	.83	- .49
Mother Vocalize --> Infant Smile	1.04	-2.97**	1.00	+ .23	1.35	+3.51***
Mother Touch --> Infant Vocalize	.72	- .84	.60	+ .05	.83	- .46
Mother Touch --> Infant Gesture	1.09	+ .69	.55	- .72	.87	-2.28
Mother Touch --> Infant Smile	.96	-2.19	.65	+ .59	2.70	-7.69***

Note: a. Contingent probability of target behaviour following criterion behaviour, lagged from the onset of the criterion behaviour across a series of 10 2-second lags.

Note: b. Magnitude $= \sum_{1}^{n} |z| / n$

Note: c. Zsum $= \sum_{1}^{n} z / \sqrt{n}$

** p ≤ .01 (two-tailed)
*** p ≤ .001 (two-tailed)

The lower half of Table 11.5 displays Z_{sums} and Magnitudes for the contingent probabilities of three infant behaviours (Vocalization, Gesture and Smile) following Maternal Vocalization and Maternal Touch. Only four of the displayed Z_{sums} are significant beyond the .01 level, and two of these are negative, implying an inhibition of the contingent infant behaviour. The pattern of infant behaviours following Maternal Vocalization is of particular interest. Following Maternal Vocalization, the Magnitudes for Infant Smile were uniformly greater than for Infant Vocalization or Gesture, indicating that the Smile is the most likely response to Maternal Vocalization. Furthermore, the Magnitudes for Infant Vocalization were uniformly lower than those for either Smile or Gesture following Maternal Vocalization.

These temporal functions demonstrate two important anomalies in the observed mother-infant interaction patterns. First, in terms of direction of effects, it is clear that the infants (admittedly unintentionally) achieved a great deal of control over their mother's behaviour, while the reverse was not true. Stated in other words, the mothers were much more responsive than their infants. Second, the lack of mutual responsiveness involving vocal behaviour contrasts sharply with the conversational quality of vocal exchanges found in sighted mother-infant dyads (Bateson, 1975). The lack of responsivity of Infant Vocalizations is surprising, given the fact that strong emphasis was placed on the reinforcement of vocalizations in the home programmes recommended to the infants' parents. Perhaps the deviation in vocal behaviour reflects differences in temporal organization rather than in rate of production. These infants did not seem to vocalize when they were expected to - neither in response to maternal behaviour nor to stimulation. Indeed, the mothers' attempts to encourage vocalization were often met with silence.

Silence, or listening, should be an especially important behaviour for a blind infant. First, auditory information is virtually the only information available about the environment that exists beyond arm's reach of the non-ambulatory blind infant. Second, it is very difficult to process competing auditory information. Listening may be so critical to the interpretation of the distal environment that it would be maladaptive for the blind infant to clutter the auditory environment with her own vocalizations. Thus, when the mother vocalizes, the infant's undivided attention, reflected by silence, may be

127

the safest response. Solitary situations, on the other hand, when the environment does not require close attention, may be 'safer' situations for vocalizing. Significantly, all three infants were reported to vocalize at a high rate when left alone.

Pragmatic Perspective

In addition to the microanalysis described above, a more global assessment of the infants' pre-verbal behaviours was achieved through the pre- and post-project administration of the maternal interview devised by Bates et al. (1977). This interview documents the presence or absence of gestural communicative behaviours as well as play, imitation and language skills.

Table 11.6 presents the pre- and post-project communicative skills for the three subjects. Clearly all three subjects displayed most of the normal mechanisms for expressing pleasure and displeasure. They also engaged in some vocal imitation and developed limited receptive vocabularies. In addition, all infants displayed repertoires of non-conventional idiosyncratic manual gestures, most of which were associated with affective states. However, only Maria began to produce words spontaneously and communicatively and only Maria produced any conventional gestures. These conventional gestures, however, developed as tricks. They were prompted by commands from adults (*Wave bye-bye* and she would wave; *Are you hungry?* and she would rub her tummy). The gestures were invariably rewarded with laughter and praise - but they were neither spontaneous nor clearly referential.

Many schemes apparently associated with language development in normal children were absent. Bates et al. (1977) had found that combinatorial and symbolic play were highly correlated with the gestural complex. Only Tanya displayed true combinatorial play and none of the infants engaged in symbolic play. A delay in symbolic play would be expected given the self/other confusion typical of visually-impaired children (Fraiberg and Adelson, 1973). Giving and showing, which normally form the basis of the early games and turn-taking rituals that Bruner (1974/5) considers precursors to the joint regulation of verbal exchanges, were virtually absent in these subjects. Only Maria had started giving by the end of the project.

Table 11.6: Pre- and Post-Project Scores on Communicative
Skills Interview[a]

Pre- and Post-Project Ages:	Amy 0;10	Amy 1;4	Maria 1;2	Maria 1;9	Tanya 1;4	Tanya 1;10
Gestural Communication						
Points						
Shows						
Gives				X		
Expresses Desire:						
Cries/Whines	X	X			X	X
Agitates					X	X
Reaches		X	X	X	X	X
Special Sound	X	X	X	X		
Word				X		
Moves to Object				X		
Expresses Dislike:						
Cries/Fusses	X	X	X	X	X	X
Agitates		X				
Special Sound		X			X	X
Pushes Away		X			X	X
Averts Head		X			X	X
Shakes Head				X		
Word				X		
Shows Off			X	X		?
Laughs with Others	X	X	X	X	X	X
Repeats Behaviour for Laughter				X	X	X
Non-conventional Gestures[b] in Filmed Sequences	9	24	13	18	4	47
Conventional Gestures[b]	0	0	2	12	0	0
Play/Imitation:						
Likes Music			X	X	X	X
Dances to Music				X		
Sings to Music			X	X		
Combinatorial Play				?	?	X
Pretends						
Imitates Vocalization		?	X	X	X	X
Imitates Gestures			X	X	?	X
Imitates Activities			X	X	?	X
Games Played[b]	0	0	5	10	2	5

Table 11.6 (cont'd)

Pre- and Post-Project Ages:	Amy 0;10	Amy 1;4	Maria 1;2	Maria 1;9	Tanya 1;4	Tanya 1;10
Language						
Understands "no"			X	X	X	X
Responds to "where is"			X	X		X
Responds to "go find"				X		
Excitement Response to Pleasant Words			X	X	X	X
Negative Response to Unpleasant Words				X		X
Touches Named Item			X	X		
Words Comprehended[b]	0	3	10	60	5	9
Words Spontaneously[b] Produced	0	0	10	42	0	0

Note: a. adapted from Bates et al. (1977).
Note: b. pre-score includes different gestures produced in four films from first observation; post-score includes all new gestures produced in subsequent films.

Pointing (an especially good predictor of language development according to Bates et al. (1977)), and reaching-as-a-request, which are both visually-guided behaviours, were of course also absent.

Both Mulford (Chapter 9) and Urwin (Chapter 13) discussed the difficulty in directing another person's attention to a distal object without the benefit of the non-verbal mechanisms available to the sighted child. Parallel to Mulford's observations on the establishment of reference, it was noted in this study that the capacity to direct attention to self developed first. All three infants were capable of attracting attention to themselves, but none of them were capable of intentionally direction attention. Thus, once the attention of the mother had been attracted, it was up to the mother to initiate the 'topic' or content of an interaction. Once her mother initiated an interaction, Maria was then able to sustain it through a series of 'turns' in a typical turn-taking routine. Amy and Tanya, however, would fill only the first turn, and then would stop. They did not seem to be able to maintain an interactive ritual, but had to be primed for each turn.

DISCUSSION

Bates et al. (1977) suggest that the gestural complex involves the use of conventional signals that have communicative function and external reference. Perhaps the absence of conventional gestural performatives in these visually-impaired subjects reflects delayed acquisition of the construct of external reference. Studies of the cognitive development of blind children (Kephart, Kephart and Schwarz, 1974; Hartlage, 1976; Lopata and Pasnak, 1976) suggest that cognitive delays may reflect experiential deficits secondary to blindness, rather than visual deprivation per se. One source of experiential deficit that may be assumed to impact seriously on cognitive and language development is the substantial lag in locomotor abilities often suffered by blind children. The pre-mobile sighted child may passively observe and absorb the concepts of self, other, agent, action, object and the relationships between them. The pre-mobile blind child has difficulty determining where she ends and another person or object begins; she may not realize that another entity exists at all if it is beyond arm's reach or if it is silent. Self/other confusion and delayed person- and object-permanence no doubt impact seriously on the acquisition of distal referencing abilities. It seems logical that the blind infant would require more active, exploratory experiences which are dependent upon an advanced level of locomotor ability to acquire the concepts and relationships critical to dual-orientation and to the establishment of distal or joint reference. I would suggest that Maria's relatively advanced locomotor abilities were critical to her advanced abilities in cognitive and communicative areas.

Just as in motor development, the blind child often goes directly from sitting to walking, unable to explore the distal environment at all until posturally mature enough to walk, so she seems to make a leap in communicative development, going directly to language as the first means of distal reference. Coordinating an unseen and unreachable adult with an unseen and unreachable object would be difficult without at least primitive referencing strategies. With neither conventional indicating gestures nor visual regard as an early means of distal reference, it becomes even more critical that early vocalizations be consistently reinforced and shaped - first into conversational patterns and eventually into language.

The uncommunicative quality of the vocal patterns observed in these three blind infants may reflect their mother's weak responses to their vocalizations. A consistent maternal response to infant vocalizations seemed to be lacking in the environments observed in this project. Given that vocal-verbal behaviour will probably be the first recognizably referential behaviour available to a blind child, close attention should be paid to the patterning of parental vocalizations and responses to infant vocalizations as a potential intervention strategy. Specific clinical recommendations for such a programme will be included in a forthcoming paper.

NOTES

1. The data were originally analyzed in three phases, each phase representing two month's worth of data per subject. The data presented here are collapsed across all three phases due to space limitations. Statements that appear in the Results section hold true when data is considered on a phase-by-phase basis as well as when collapsed across phases.

Chapter 12.

COGNITION, INTERACTION, AND DEVELOPMENT, WITH SPE-
CIAL REFERENCE TO EDUCATION OF THE HANDICAPPED CHILD

Ton van der Geest

INTRODUCTION

In her paper Charity Rowland (Chapter 11) is mainly
concerned with the presentation and discussion of
the results of her investigation into mother-blind
child interaction. She did not consider more theoretical and practical matters concerning interaction, language acquisition, and education. I will
try therefore to address the context and type of
problems in which the investigation of mother-child
interaction, and in this special case the interaction between blind children and their mothers, makes
sense. Rowland's work illustrates some of the problems typical of interaction research which I would
like to discuss further. I will also present some
opinions on the question of how to put into practice
the results of language acquisition research.

LANGUAGE ACQUISITION AND MOTHER-CHILD INTERACTION

Three theories of language acquisition have been recently discussed in depth by Clahsen (1981). The
first theory he treats is based on universal grammar. Within this theory it is essential that the
child have an innate mechanism at his disposal that
determines the form of a possible human language and
furthermore an evaluation yard-stick by which the
child is able to select that grammar that is both
compatible with the primary linguistic data and as
simple as possible (mentalistic theory). Interactive theory, the second treated, holds that the
acquisition of syntax is significantly influenced by
the form of verbal interactions between child and
mother. The third theory Clahsen discusses is cognitive theory. Certain cognitive operations are

here a condition for the acquisition of language.
Linguistic learning processes are essentially determined by the cognitive complexity of the linguistic
structures to be learned.

Mentalistic linguistic theory is rejected by
Clahsen on, in my opinion, valid grounds and I refer
to his work for the detailed arguments. The interactive theory can only be accepted in so far as
mother-child interaction is one of the essential
conditions that enable the child to acquire his language. It is to be rejected - as Clahsen argues -
since this approach does not explain the learning
processes that lead to the acquisition of syntax.
This problem can, according to Clahsen, probably
only be resolved by the cognitive theory as deduced
from Piaget's theory (Sinclair, 1970) and as worked
out by Slobin (1973).

Apart from the question whether Clahsen's evaluation of the theories is correct or not, it is
clear that the study of mother-child interaction can
be motivated extrinsically. An analysis of this
interaction can be of great help in those cases in
which languages may develop deviantly, especially
where the child is handicapped with deafness or
blindness. Since the quality of the primary linguistic data at least determines to a very large extent how prosperously language develops, it can be
concluded that actual knowledge of mother-child
interaction, in the case of both the normal and the
handicapped child, can be applied in order to influence development positively.

Clahsen's rejection of the interactive theory
can also be questioned. Firstly, he does not himself investigate mother-child interaction but only
the development of syntactic complexity in child utterances. So his conclusions are based only on the
literature referred to in his discussion of the theories.

Secondly, it has been shown that cognitive complexity is <u>not fully independent</u> of the way in which
mothers and children interact, for example in the
work by Brown and Hanlon (1970), Bruner (1974/5),
Miller (1976), Van der Geest (1977, 1978), Miller
and Weissenborn (1979) and Van der Geest and
Heckhausen (1981).

Thirdly, it must be emphasized here that it is
not necessarily correct to assume that one theory
alone must be able to explain such complex processes
as those underlying language acquisition. It is,
for example, easy to see that, in more than one respect, cognitive and interactive theory may be

complementary. If we accept, for example, that a cognitive theory of language acquisition must be based on Piaget's theory of intellectual development, then we have to accept not only the cognitive processes within the child's mind (the child's activity) but also the interactive aspect of Piaget's theory in which it is emphasized that what the child learns is the product of the interaction between the active child and his environment. This implies that how the child's environment is structured is one of the two relevant factors of development. Furthermore, it can be shown that the cognitive prerequisites in the child's development are directly correlated with the linguistic structuring of the dialogue by the mother. This means, in my opinion, that mother-child interaction is not only one of the essential conditions for language acquisition but also is intrinsically relevant to the processes of language acquisition itself.

Rowland's paper may illustrate this relevance. She reports some remarkable differences between mother-child interaction dependent on whether the child develops well or not. The infant behaviours "non-vocal sound", "manipulate toy", and "reach for toy" and the mother behaviours "vocalization" are positively related to development. The proportions of intervals for these variables reflect fully the development of the three children Rowland investigated (see Table 11.3). The infant behaviours "touch self" and "no manual activity" and mother behaviours "touch" and "non-vocal sound" are negatively related to child development. There are, furthermore, some interesting differences in the interactions. In the prosperous interaction, there are not only systematic mother reactions to the child's vocalizations which are absent in the other interactions, but there is also a systematic child reaction to the mother's vocalizations in the well-developed interaction. I do, however, miss a discussion of the impacts of these relevant results in Rowland's paper.

METHODOLOGY OF THE INVESTIGATION OF MOTHER-CHILD INTERACTION

In interaction and communicative research, both category systems and sign systems can be applied. If nothing or relatively little is known about the topic, than a sign system should be applied. In such a system as many aspects as possible are investigated;

instead of categories of aspects, elementary aspects should be investigated. In this way one is able to deduce what kinds of aspects are relevant for the topic under investigation and what aspects can be grouped into one category. Thereafter category systems can be applied in order to have a larger amount of data pertinent to the individual variables. Linguists prefer working with sign systems. Labov and Fanshel's (1977) work is a good example in this respect for showing how such initial detecting work proceeds. Social psychologists normally prefer category systems but this is not only based on previous work with sign systems but in fact mostly on intuition.

Although a lot of research on mother-child interaction has been done in the last five years, we have to admit that still only a little is known about how they actually interact. The results of most studies reveal only that interaction is relevant to language development, not, however, the form interaction takes and how it influences language acquisition. There are a few exceptions (e.g. Van der Geest, 1977) but such studies can be criticized on other grounds (see Brown, 1977; McTear, 1978). The main objection to my paper concerns the 'direct observation - indirect interpretation' controversy as discussed for example by Fiske (1978) and Van der Geest (1981). In almost all experimentally, psychometrically and statistically oriented designs, the direct observations are not described; instead, only an interpretation of the results of statistical analysis is given. Only when the observation of interaction is reported, are we able to examine whether two subsequent actions of two partners are related to each other or are independent, and, if they are related, on what level.

Relations between two events that are in principle independent, cannot be determined through statistical analysis. We can only infer that a relation may exist between two types of events. This is essentially what McTear (1978) criticizes in my paper. Especially in cases in which we are trying to discover regularities first or to detect the central variables in a new area of research, it makes sense to restrict one's activities initially to mere observation. As I have already mentioned, the study of mother-child interaction with respect to language acquisition is still in its infancy. This is even more the case for the study of special cases of interaction involving, for example, blind or deaf children. For deaf children I know of only one

observational study (Tervoort, 1981); for blind children Rowland's study is the only one to my knowledge. The state of the art of interaction research with respect to language development has to lead, in my opinion, automatically to observational research. These two points, that is that, at least at the initial stage of research, (1) category systems should be avoided, and (2) observational, rather than statistical studies should be carried out, will be discussed in more detail in relation to work with blind children.

Category Systems

Concerning the behavioural variables used in the analysis, it can be deduced from the section "Procedures and Analysis" that Rowland used a category system: 7 child-behaviour categories, 3 mother-behaviour categories, and a total of 42 subcategories. As neither categories nor subcategories are mentioned in the text, we may only guess that they have been extracted from interaction research with the sighted child. This is, however, problematic for more than one reason. Besides the fact that postulated categories in new research areas should be avoided, in this very special case we must determine whether the categories of interaction with the sighted child, are relevant for interaction with blind children. The results of Rowland's study are already evidence enough to conclude that there are systematic differences between these two types of interaction.

This conclusion may also be the solution to the problem in Piagetian theory with respect to cognitive development in the sighted, deaf and blind child. From Furth (1966) and Oléron (1957) it is clear that deaf children develop almost normally. This is in sharp contrast to cognitive development in the blind child, which, at least at the transitional stage from pre- to concrete operations, is enormously (almost four years) retarded (Hatwell, 1960, as cited in Sinclair de Zwart, 1969). If it is accepted from both Piagetian research and from research in language acquisition (e.g. Clahsen, 1981) that cognition is a kind of pace-maker for language acquisition, it follows necessarily that for blind children there must be an enormous delay in language development. This does not, however, always appear to be the case, as may be evident from the blind child, Maria, in Rowland's data and from the work of Urwin (1978b), and Fraiberg (1977). We are,

therefore, in the awkward situation of looking for
an explanation of this Piagetian paradox. An explanation that would make sense is to assume that cognitive development in the blind and normal child
takes different routes. The assumption is plausible
if we allow that cognitive development is a result
of interaction between the active child and its environment and that the quality of the blind child's
environment is essentially different from that of
the sighted child. The delay found in the cognitive
development of the blind child, may be nothing more
than an artifact of the false assumption that blind
children develop cognitively along the same routes
as sighted children. If it is assumed that they develop along different routes and that cognition is a
necessary prerequisite of language acquisition, we
may conclude that different aspects of communicative
behaviour are relevant to investigation. It is
therefore questionable whether the categories in
Rowland's study are fully adequate for the problem
she investigated.

Observational vs. Statistical Analysis

Rowland draws conclusions with respect to interaction on the basis of statistical analysis, instead
of on the basis of observation. If I understand
Rowland correctly, she analyzed the supplement behaviours of mother and child in order to conclude
whether a type of sequence (e.g. A,B) occurred more
frequently than can be expected on the basis of
probability. It was not investigated whether or not
in each occurrence behaviour A and behaviour B were
interrelated in substance.

On the contrary, she accepted as subsequent behaviour a behaviour that occurred as much as 20 seconds later (more or less the time span an athlete
needs to cover 200 yards). It is also allowed that,
between A and B, other behaviours that are relevant
for the interaction analysis occurred. Even if this
is not the case, the problem remains unsolved whether A and B are only subsequent to each other or
whether they are interdependent. It is unclear
whether coincidental events should be regarded as
systematic or not. In my opinion the statistical
procedure of 'lagging' leads to severe problems in
interpretation, since it implies that behaviours
which are subsequent to one another also interact
with one another (see title of Rowland's paper).

Another methodological point concerns the fact
that the same categories are used not only for three

children that are very different from each other in terms of development, but also for the same child during six months of observation. From the description of the children and from Table 11.3, it appears that the three children developed rather well during this period so that we may guess that other types of behaviours came into the foreground. By this very fact some effects of interaction and development may become invisible if the frequencies that are analyzed statistically concern the number of occurrences in the data of the whole period.

A longitudinal investigation of mother-child interaction has confirmed this point. Twelve children were studied in the age range from 1;0 to 2;1 (Van der Geest and Nörenberg, in prep.). In this investigation we subdivided the children into two groups: six quick and six slow developers, and looked for interactive differences between the two groups. We found that (1) different communicative variables played a role in the adaptation of the mother to the child's communicative level in the two groups; (2) children 'preferred' different variables in their communications with their mothers; (3) many variables described in earlier investigations did not discriminate between the two groups of interactions; (4) only after a division of the children into four groups and analysing each session separately were we able to demonstrate that linguistic variables are only discriminating with respect to mothers' adaptation and children's preferent usage during a very short time span. I hope that such developmental questions as raised here will be answered in the (planned) fuller publication of Rowland's investigations.

ADAPTABILITY OF MOTHERS

Apart from these critical remarks, with respect to research methodology, we can say that many of the results and interpretations of these results are interesting for the description of communicative development in blind children. The results show that there are obviously great differences between interactions with sighted and with blind children; and that these differences can not only be explained as delay; the high rates of touching and reactions of the mothers to the infant smile seem worthwhile mentioning here. As can also be observed in mother-sighted child interaction, the infants affected their mothers' behaviour much more strongly and

systematically than the mothers affected the infant's behaviour. I would interpret this fact rather as an adaptive quality of the mother than as an influencing capacity of the child. It is the child's contribution to produce those behaviours that are attractive for the mother to react to. It is the mother's creative contribution to pick up on this child activity and to reinforce it by appropriate communications and reactions. The fact that the child does not react so often can perhaps be explained by the fact that (1) the child does not have a teaching task; (2) the child has only a very small reaction repertoire at his disposal; (3) reacting is much more difficult than behaving if the context is not restricted by ongoing interaction.

FURTHER RESEARCH

Before any conclusions are drawn for educational programmes with the blind, a more detailed description is necessary of interaction in mother-blind child pairs. I can only repeat my belief that a more observational approach would have been more effective in describing the interactional and developmental processes adequately, and that only on the basis of such observational data can therefore well founded recommendations for intervention be made. Prevalent clinical practice leads me to fear that statistically established categories will lead to the setting up of diagnostic tests and on these tests recommendations for intervention and treatment will be based. This is common practice, although tests measure the products and not the processes leading to these products and therefore do not deliver indications for treatment of the individual case. In my opinion, shared also by Fiske (1978), it is better to investigate behaviour with a minimum of postulates and theory and to find out what kinds of behaviours are critical. Instead of applying tests, one should diagnose by the observation of behaviour (with the help of critical variables) because observation leads to knowledge of the facts, the underlying processes, and the system. Instead of a standardized programme we need an intervention method to influence the processes of the system.
    In order to come to grips with what is going on in mother-blind child interaction and with the question of how cognition and language develops in a sightless child, the basic investigation of interaction between a blind child and a blind mother may be

of great help, especially in so far as diagnosis and intervention are concerned. The argumentation with respect to this belief must, unfortunately, be indirect, and derives from research with the deaf child.

From many investigations with deaf children (e.g. Tervoort, 1972) it appears that congenitally deaf children who have deaf parents have generally greater language capacity in both the deaf's sign language and in the oral language of the environment than deaf children with hearing parents. One could argue that deaf parents have a better understanding of the deaf child's communicative problems and will be, therefore, more efficient language trainers with respect to the language acquisition of the deaf than hearing parents are. It would make sense, therefore, to investigate this typical interaction and this typical language development in order to detect how the language learner situation is structured optimally and how parents interact optimally with respect to development. It seems reasonable to me that the same would apply to the blind child.

Chapter 13.

DIALOGUE AND COGNITIVE FUNCTIONING IN THE EARLY LAN-
GUAGE DEVELOPMENT OF THREE BLIND CHILDREN

Cathy Urwin

Like several contributions to this volume, this
chapter is about the earliest stages of language acquisition, and the developments which enable blind
children to use language in the first place.   It
presents findings from an intensive longitudinal
study of three congentially blind infants (Urwin,
1978a), with the aim of challenging two assumptions
which are frequently made about blind children's development.   The first of these is that certain aspects of development, in language and cognition, are
necessarily delayed in blind children.   The second
is that acquiring language is relatively 'unhelpful'
in the development of cognitive functioning.   Finally, the chapter probes the question of how far, if
at all, studying blind children's language development can throw light on the normal process.

RECENT RESEARCH INTO LANGUAGE ACQUISITION IN SIGHTED
CHILDREN

My starting point is recent work with sighted children which has been discussed or referred to elsewhere in this volume (e.g. in Mills' introduction,
and in the contributions from Rowland and Van der
Geest).   This work argues for a relationship between
infant development and the earliest stages of language acquisition, and very broadly can be divided
into two major lines of approach.   One has concentrated on semantic aspects of language and proposes
that cognitive schemes established in infancy provide the conceptual input for children's earliest
utterances (e.g. Bowerman, 1973; Brown, 1973;
Edwards, 1973; Nelson, 1973).   Here, probably the
most influential approaches have drawn on Piaget's
(1951, 1953, 1955) theory, to argue, for example

that the development of sensorimotor intelligence contributes to constraints on the kinds of words acquired through the single word stage and to systematic changes in their usage (Bloom, 1973), and that its terminal achievements account for apparent universals in the conceptual relations underlying the first word combinations (Bowerman, 1973; Brown, 1973; Edwards, 1973; Slobin, 1973).

The other major line of approach has been primarily concerned with communication and functional aspects of language, and has aimed to demonstrate a developmental continuity between pre-verbal and verbal communication, for example by Bates, Camaioni and Volterra (1975), Bruner (1975, 1978), Carter (1974, 1978), and Halliday (1975). Here, the theoretical frameworks have been far more diverse, varying from applications of different versions of Speech Act Theory (Bates et al., 1975; Bruner, 1975), through Halliday's (1973, 1975) own functional theory, to Carter's (1974, 1978) descriptive study of the evolution of one child's gestural communication system. There are a number of unresolved problems with this work, some of which centre around moving beyond speculation or reasoning-by-analogy in accounting for the origins of syntactic structure in communicative terms (for critiques, see, for example, Schaffer, 1977; Dore, 1978). But as far as the initial entry into language is concerned, the concensus is sufficient to establish that, before they begin to speak, sighted children have already consolidated simple communicative procedures for initiating interaction, making demands and directing the behaviour and attention of others. Once they begin to acquire standard words, these procedures persist as accompaniments to children's early utterances, and serve to convey the particular communicative effects which they intend (Carter, 1974; Bates et al., 1975; Bruner, 1975, 1978; Dore, 1975). Thus, the communicative functions first expressed with words are related to those already available to the child, a finding which is taken to endorse the general notion that the "very nature" of the child's pre-speech communication system may be such as to aid the passage through to language (Bruner, 1978).

IMPLICATIONS FOR BLIND CHILDREN

Now whether one emphasizes the propositional content of children's utterances or the communicative functions served by using them, both these lines of

143

approach lead to the prediction that blindness will pose considerable problems for infant development and that this will have consequences for the emergence of language. Piaget's theory, for example, on which many semantic approaches have relied, is often interpreted as giving vision a primary role (Cromer, 1973), and indeed Piaget's own writings imply that lack of vision will "slow down" cognitive development in infancy (Piaget and Inhelder, 1969). If this view is correct, we might anticipate that blind children will be initially delayed in acquiring words and in forming word combinations, and/or there will be restrictions in underlying meaning relations in both the single word period and afterwards (see Landau (Chapter 7) and Werth (Chapter 8)).

But the sighted child literature predicts perhaps even greater constraints on blind children's learning to use language to communicate. Despite their differing theoretical frameworks, the majority of pre-verbal communication studies in sighted children have concentrated on just those communication systems which blind children lack. These include the use of eye-to-eye contact in the regulation of early reciprocal exchanges between mother and child (Bruner, 1975; see also Brazelton, Koslowski and Main, 1974; Stern, 1974), the use of the visual system in monitoring mutual attention to distal objects and events, a capacity which is said to provide the basis for establishing a shared frame of reference (Bruner, 1975, 1978; see also Collis and Schaffer, 1975), and the use of gestures such as indicative pointing and reaching-in-demand. Along with 'showing off' to gain adult attention and 'give and take games' with objects, these gestural procedures typically emerge in the last quarter of the first year (Carter, 1974; Bates et al., 1975; Bruner, 1975, 1978; see also Trevarthen and Hubley, 1978). The availability of these procedures is assumed to contribute to what are dominant language functions in many sighted children in the early stages, using words to name and to make requests for objects. Thus one would again expect that the absence of these and other visually-based communication means would delay the onset of language, and/or restrict the kinds of communicative functions which blind children are able to express.

If we look at the available evidence on blind children's development there is apparently considerable support for these predictions. The work of Fraiberg (1977), Adelson (Chapter 1) and other clinical investigators (e.g. Burlingham, 1961, 1964;

Wills, 1970), emphasizes the severe problems which blindness poses for development in infancy, in both cognitive functioning and social interaction. Although clinicians and educators are well aware of the relatively high incidence of language problems among school-age blind children (see Urwin, 1978b; Elstner, Chapter 3), up until now there has been surprisingly little work on the language of younger children. But what evidence there is suggests that problems with semantic and/or communicative aspects of language are extremely common, even in children for whom there is no reason to suspect additional neurological damage. For example, many blind children are initially delayed in acquiring their first words, and may not immediately use them spontaneously in communication. They may repeat them to themselves in their own play, and fail to produce them to initiate interaction, requiring some prompt to imitate on the part of the parent until well into the third year (Wood, 1970). Though other children acquire their first words within the sighted age range, social words and phrases often markedly predominate over words for referring to objects, such that the children appear to be showing an extreme form of a language acquisition strategy which, for sighted children, Nelson (1973) has characterized as "expressive". In some cases the child's language may remain tied to his or her body movement or to familiar social routines for a prolonged period, and a reliance on phrases acquired wholesale is often coupled with a marked propensity for imitation and/or echolalia. Even the group studied by Fraiberg (1977) and Adelson (Chapter 1), who had the advantage of clinical intervention, showed some delay in using words to name objects and in the production of the first word combinations. These delays, Fraiberg and Adelson suggest, were due to constraints on the development of sensorimotor intelligence and the emergence of representation in the Piagetian sense, the latter being delayed in all the children in the sample.

This position is consistent with the semantic approaches to sighted child language discussed above, and concentrates on the origins of the propositional content of children's utterances. But naming objects is generally, of course, also a communicative act, frequently accompanied by gesture in sighted children. Blind children do not, apparently, point spontaneously to distant objects. This raises the question of the implications of the absence of particular pre-verbal procedures.

Consistent with this, there is evidence suggesting that the use of words to make requests, particularly for objects, is slow to emerge in blind children. Wills' (personal communication) observations, for example, suggest that requests based on internal need states, such as demands for food or body action, are likely to emerge considerably earlier than demands for things in the external world. This would again support the assumption that young blind children are constrained by the absence of gesturing in the pre-verbal period and/or by lack of knowledge of the permanent existence of objects. In addition, there is one developmental delay which Adelson (Chapter 1) and Fraiberg (Fraiberg and Adelson, 1975; Fraiberg, 1977) have proposed is universal in blind children: a delay in the acquisition of I as a stable pronoun and, by implication, the ability to use you to refer to the other party in interaction. Fraiberg and Adelson propose that this delay is related to a delay in a more general developmental process, the capacity for self representation. Pronominal reference is, of course, a later development than the ones discussed so far. But the claim is nonetheless in line with the assumption that blindness inhibits the development of reciprocal interaction and/or independent action in infancy, and that this has cumulative implications for language development.

Broadly speaking, then, these observations are consistent with predictions drawn from the sighted child literature. They would thus seem to support the theoretical assumptions underlying that work, and the priority it explicitly or implicitly assumes for vision. But for children who do not have vision, it would be an extremely negative conclusion to leave the matter there. It is all too easy to assume that difficulties are an inevitable consequence of blindness. Furthermore, there are many dangers in relying entirely on theories of sighted children's development in understanding the development of blind children.

Firstly, the theories of 'normal' development with which one begins may be wrong or in some ways inadequate, even in their own terms. For example, there is currently considerable dissatisfaction with the way Piaget's theory has been applied to the study of language acquisition in sighted children (see, for example, McShane, 1980; Elliot, 1981), and the theory itself is increasingly being criticized for its neglect of social aspects of cognition (see Donaldson, 1978; Walkerdine and Sinha, 1978;

146

Walkerdine and Corran, 1979). Secondly, if a theory
of 'normal' development already gives priority to
vision, then that theory itself cannot tell us what
alternative routes may be available to blind children, nor what form adaptation to the absence of vision might take. Nor will it explain why common
'anomalies' should take the particular form that
they do.

To answer these questions we have to uncover
the processes of adaptive development. This may
best be achieved by taking a closer look at what
blind children actually do. The next section describes the development of three congentially blind
children whose language and overall development has
progressed extremely well, even when compared to the
children in Fraiberg's sample. This provides an opportunity for demonstrating what can be achieved by
blind children, questioning many assumptions as to
the necessity of developmental delay. In itself
this may have important implications for the kinds
of guidance which it is appropriate to give to parents of other blind children. But in so far as
these children's development contradicts the predictions drawn from the theories of development in
sighted children, we may also be required to reexam-
ine the adequacy of these theories, even for sighted
children.

A LONGITUDINAL STUDY

The three children are all legally blind and have no
additional neurological damage. Jerry and Suzanne
are both totally blind through optic atrophy, but
Steven has a little sight in one eye, in which he
has glaucoma and aniridia. Though extremely limited, this vision gave Steven considerable advantages.
Nevertheless his early communicative behaviour and
language showed many characteristics differentiating
him from fully sighted children.

The three children were observed, video- and
audio-recorded in the home in interaction with one
or other of their parents at regular intervals. The
research methods, described more fully elsewhere
(see Urwin, 1978a), included a descriptive analysis
of the development of communicative exchange between
each mother-child pair, and a longitudinal analysis
of each mother's own use of speech. By and large,
cognitive development was assessed through observations of the children's spontaneous play with objects. Jerry and Steven were followed through a

large part of the pre-verbal period and the one-word stage to the point at which they began producing their first combinations. The studies were closed at approximately 20 months in both cases. Suzanne was followed through the first 14 months by Dr. Michael Tobin who has made his video- and other records available to me. I myself began following Suzanne when she was 15 months old, and made monthly recordings until 22 months. Further extended recording sessions took place at two years and two years three months. Unlike Steven and Jerry, who are both first born children, Suzanne has a sister, Elaine, who is two years older and sighted. Elaine was present for a large part of each recording session.

The relatively satisfactory development of these children, when compared to that of the blind child population as a whole, was largely due to the opportunities for social interaction and active exploration provided by the parents. Though there were considerable differences in the children's home environments and in the parents' beliefs about children's development (see Urwin, 1978c), the interactions between the three children and their parents nevertheless had many features in common. Of these, the most crucial concerned the extent to which all the parents made use of non-visual communication systems themselves, and discovered alternative cues to the infants' attention, involvement and intention.

In the early months, for example, in spite of the absence of or (in Steven's case) reduced eye-contact, all the mothers would watch their babies' faces intently, 'mirroring' changes of facial expression and the effect of body movement in their voices. They also used touching, stroking, tickling and grosser forms of body play extensively, elaborating their own routines or adapting versions of well known games such as "pat-a-cake", "ride-a-cock horse" and even "peekaboo". As I have described elsewhere (Urwin, 1978c), the parents would use the predictability inherent in these games to build up expectancies, encourage anticipation, and eventually to 'push' the babies towards taking more active roles. By the end of the first year all three infants were capable of dictating the 'next step' in these games, using their own bodies to control their parents' actions and reactions, and accompanying these procedures with distinctive prosodic marking.

Vocalization, too, was another area which these parents encouraged. In all three cases the mothers

would not only talk to their infants, but also mark, question, imitate or otherwise respond to their babies' pre-verbal vocalizations, prompting them to vocalize in turn. In contrast to some of the mother-child pairs described by Rowland (Chapter 11), by the last quarter of the first year each of these infants would collaborate in and prolong vocal imitation sequences and quasi-dialogues, the children showing an exquisite control over the adults' following responses (see Urwin, 1979). Jerry, for example, would keep in contact with his mother for as long as 20 minutes at a time while she got on with the housework in the next-door room.

Despite the absence of vision, these children thus showed an ability to allocate 'turns' in interaction (see McGurk, Chapter 10), and to control the other's actions which was well on a par with sighted children. Their ability to manage body-play routines, for example, emerged over the age range when sighted children begin to 'show off' to court adult attention and to use gestures (Bates et al., 1975), and may thus be regarded as parallel developments. In the emergence of language and its early development, similarities with sighted children were again striking. As is consistent with the evidence discussed above on continuity of a function between pre-verbal and verbal communication in sighted children, each of the children's early words used in communication were initially accompanied by pre-existing vocal and/or action procedures which conveyed particular communicative intentions. These included demands for body-action, protests or requests that a particular game be repeated, and in the vocal sphere the pre-verbal vocal 'dialoguing' paved the way for an unusually early mastery of basic conversation-maintaining procedures. These included the use of rising intonation to prompt replies and various devices for opening and closing encounters (Sachs, Schegloff and Jefferson, 1974; Urwin, 1979). As for the children's lexical development, in each case their first words originated in affective or routinized interaction contexts in which he or she had gained some measure of active control. Again this is typical of many sighted children (see, for example, the data reported by Bowerman, 1978 and Ferrier, 1978). Though not all kinds of over-extensions observable in sighted children could be identified (see Urwin, 1979) through the single-word period, these children nevertheless extended early acquired words into new contexts including those involving objects, thus shifting the locus away from

their own bodies. At around 18 months their vocabularies expanded rapidly and they began to produce their first word combinations. In each case these developments occurred with the beginnings of pretend play and changes in search behaviour which indicated that the children knew of the continued existence of objects apart from their own actions and independent of specific locations.

Such close parallels with sighted children's developments clearly challenge the assumption that the emergence of representation is necessarily delayed in blind children. However, it was not the case that there were no areas of relative restriction for these children. For example, since they could not look towards their mothers, before the emergence of language their ability to initiate interaction was somewhat restricted. Thus the play exchanges described above still depended on physical contact up to the end of the first year, and hence on the parents' prior decisions to put themselves at their infants' disposal. Limitations in the means available to the blind infants to initiate interaction have been commented on by Fraiberg (1977), and Wills (1970). But for these children, situations which involved the mothers and children having to attend to distant objects and events also posed significant constraints. In this the difficulties were as great for the parents as for the children. The sighted child literature, as mentioned above, has made much of the potency of visual gaze as a cue to the child's attention to distant objects (Bruner, 1975, 1978; Collis and Schaffer, 1975). In contrast, cues associated with listening are far more ambiguous, such that it was comparatively rare for the mothers to perceive and comment on things that the infants might have been listening to unless they were producing the sounds themselves. By the same token, of course, the infants were limited in gaining access to the objects of others' attention. Similarly, where sighted children may use gestures such as reaching in demand and indicative pointing to direct attention towards distant objects, this kind of gesturing did not, apparently, emerge spontaneously in these children. Nor did they offer and exchange objects without deliberate training on the part of the parents.

Constraints on initiating interaction and on establishing mutual attention to distant objects and events at first restricted the children's use of language. For example, in the two totally blind children, using language to initiate particular

forms of play, as distinct from using it to sustain or restart some game already underway, did not emerge until well into the second year, after a period in which they learned to use movements from well established routines to control the parents' actions and reactions across the space between them. Once language began, of course, a relatively unambiguous means for initiating interaction was available to them. Perhaps related to this, by the end of the single word period all the children had amassed a large number of names of significant people. These the totally blind children used particularly frequently . Suzanne, for example, would call out to the people present and even to the children next door when she heard them playing in the street. But by the time they began to combine words, none of the children were observed producing utterances which referred explicitly to other people as agents of their own actions (as would be expressed in utterances of the form *Mummy push* or *Mummy go*, for example). This is not an early development for sighted children either, nevertheless Greenfield and Smith (1976) report that the two children in their longitudinal study had begun to refer to others' agency by the end of the single word period. Nor did the blind children comment on other people's possession of objects at this stage, though they referred to their own.

Related constraints appeared in the way these children named objects. In acquiring names of people, of course, they were acquiring words for objects which were capable of answering back. In contrast, relatively few inanimate objects in their environments produced sounds without being acted on. All three children would name familiar objects, sound-producing or otherwise, when they contacted them physically, or in Steven's case, when they came within his limited visual range. But at this time none of the children would name or refer to objects remote from themselves. Nor did they make requests for them. Steven began to demand objects at around 18 months, but these demands were restricted to particularly familiar things when he could see them. Jerry had not begun to demand objects by the close of the study. Suzanne's first requests for objects emerged at around 21 months, when they were extremely infrequent and handled with questions of the form *Where's X?*. This was in spite of the fact that a semantic analysis of her language at this time provided examples of each of the two-term semantic relations which Brown (1973) has argued are related

to, and depend on, the emergence of representation.
A superficial inspection might suggest that at
this time these children's language showed the restrictions relative to sighted children which are
common amongst the blind child population as a
whole, and which have been described above. But
here the kinds of explanations which can be derived
from the sighted child literature are of relatively
limited value. A simple explanation in terms of a
'delay' in some general cognitive process, for example is clearly inadequate for these children. Their
language development in other areas was well on a
par with that of sighted children; their search behaviour and other activities involving objects indicated that they knew of the permanent existence of
objects, and further developments in social play indicated that they had some understanding of revers-
ible roles and other people's agency (Urwin, 1978a,
1978c). Moreover it is misleading to assume that
similar functions for language, such as naming and
making requests for distant objects, necessarily represent equivalent developmental achievements in
blind and sighted children. In sighted children of
this age this behaviour is largely or entirely elicited by things which are in view or by visual props
in the immediate context, such as cues which indicate their habitual location (Huxley and Urwin, unpublished data). In contrast, blind children are
excluded from much that is going on around them.
For them to name and request objects is perhaps more
akin to sighted children's referring to things which
are absent or concealed, with the minimum support
from the immediate context. This use of language is
not observable with any degree of frequency in the
early stages, suggesting that apparently similar
phenomena may represent more complex developmental
achievements on the part of blind children.
It is in just such areas, however, that language can provide blind children with many advantages, enabling them to achieve what sighted children achieve with gesture in the pre-verbal period,
and to refer to and seek information about events to
which they have little or no direct access. But another limitation with the sighted child literature
now becomes apparent. Though the absence of some
communication system in infancy, such as the use of
gesture, may well have contributed to the blind
children's difficulties, there is nothing in that
literature which explains how these difficulties can
ever be resolved. To understand this, we again have
to look at the blind children themselves. This was

possible for Suzanne since she was followed to an older age.

SUZANNE'S LATER DEVELOPMENT

For Suzanne, the answer is somewhat paradoxical. For her the resolution of early restrictions, relative to sighted children, was greatly aided by the entry into language itself, or more properly, the opportunities which this created for dialogue with other people. Here there were a number of ways in which Suzanne's mother's own use of speech appeared particularly suited to extending the child's access to the surrounding context. This can be illustrated particularly clearly by looking at interaction sequences invovling mutual attention to objects, and at the significance of Suzanne's ability to name them for herself.

As mentioned previously, the research methods used in this study included an analysis of each mother's speech to her child. In many respects, as applied in all three cases, Suzanne's mother's speech showed just those syntactic, semantic, and functional characteristics which have now been described many times for mothers speaking to their sighted children (e.g. Snow, 1977a). In addition, her speech showed a predominance of various dialogue-sustaining devices, such as the use of expansions and incorporations, which Cross (1977) found correlated with rapid speech development in sighted children. However, there were also some significant differences, which again applied to the other two mothers. Compared to the two mothers of sighted infants studied longitudinally by Snow (1977b), these mothers talked relatively more about the 'child' and relatively less about objects and events in the 'outside world' for much of the pre-verbal period. This partly reflected the extent to which the mothers of blind children used their own speech to frame their babies' body actions and facial expressions, feeding back their effects on those who watched them, as described above. But it may also have been due to the relative paucity of cues to the blind children's attention to distant objects and events, such as looking and gesture itself.

Nevertheless, the mothers of the blind infants could refer to objects which the children were investigating close at hand. This Suzanne's mother did particularly frequently, which allowed the child to become familiar with the names of particular

objects. At the same time the process also marked
the fact that these objects were accessible to the
mother as well as to the child herself. In consequence, as soon as Suzanne began to name objects and
the mother to acknowledge this verbally, language
itself provided Suzanne with a means for establishing that her proximal space was shareable with other
people, despite her lack of vision. This change in
the child's initiatives had important implications
for changes in the mother's contribution to the interaction. Apart from the fact that she was now answering verbal initiatives, Suzanne's using object
names appropriately made it indubitably clear to the
mother that the child knew of the things to which
these words referred. Coupled with the observable
changes in Suzanne's searching for objects which occurred over the same period, this led the mother to
refer more frequently to familiar objects when they
were beyond the child's range of touch. For example, she began to use the names of familiar objects
in *Where's X?* questions to prompt the child to explore the space around her: *Where's the car?*,
Where's your dolly, Suzanne?, *Find your dolly for
Mummy*, and so on. Prompting the child's action, the
mother's language again drew attention to a shared
space. Reversing the procedure, it was this question form which the child appropriated to express
her first requests for objects.

Yet the ability to articulate demands itself
added a new dimension to the interaction. Over the
same time period, Suzanne was becoming increasingly
mobile. Besides bringing her into direct contact
with more objects which were further afield, this
also opened new contexts in which talk could take
place. Though the mother named new objects with
which the child came into contact, she became less
likely to respond to the child's requests for objects by actually providing them. Rather, she would
prompt the child to get them for herself by specifying their location relative to the child, or to familiar landmarks for which she now had names: *This
way, That way, It's on the table, It's in the bed-
room*, or *It's by the door*. Thus, by taking what the
child said as a starting point and relying on her
understanding of familiar words, the mother's language linked the child to the surrounding context.
Again the child took over many of the mother's location markers, such that she was using terms such as
in and *on* frequently and appropriately by the end of
the study, to refer to places outside her own body.

Apart from contributing to her ability to talk

about objects and locations, dialogue with her mother also facilitated Suzanne's using language to refer to other people's actions and possession of objects. Looking at the origins and emergence of Suzanne's references to her sister, Elaine, illustrates this particularly closely.

As mentioned above, Elaine was present for a large part of each recording session. During this time Suzanne's mother would consistently refer to her in her speech to Suzanne, keeping her comments within the kinds of things Suzanne was likely to understand. Increasingly these references came in response to verbal initiatives from Suzanne as, from 18 months onwards, she began to call out to her sister by name, often as she produced some sound which caught her attention. The mother would comment on what Elaine was doing, thus providing a basis from which Suzanne could interpret the significance of particular sounds. From the end of the second year the kinds of activities in which the two children engaged became more obviously similar. They played with many of the same toys, for example, such that references to Elaine in the mother's speech began to include statements or explanations about Elaine's actions on familiar objects. By the third year the mother was obliged to sort out some competition between the two sisters. Many of Suzanne's requests for objects, for example, were prompted by her recognizing what her sister was playing with, either by the sound of the thing itself, or through understanding what Elaine was saying. The following example shows how, at the close of the study, Suzanne was now using language to establish mutual attention to objects, to refer to objects distant from herself, and to distinguish her own and the other's access to them. Reconstructing the language which the mother used habitually to 'keep the peace' between the two sisters, Suzanne marks the relation of possession. Perhaps at the same time she is coming to terms with notions of sharing (Suzanne 2;3).

Example 1. Suzanne: *Elaine's got the case.*
            Mother : *Elaine's got the case, yes.*
            Suzanne: *And I got the hairdrier,*
                      naughty old hairdrier!

Suzanne's ability to refer to Elaine and her actions was, of course, related to the fact that her sister's activities were predictable and very similar to her own. Yet at the same time, though consistently drawing attention to this relationship,

the mother's language helped to provide the bridge. Once again, the use of language enabled Suzanne to penetrate contexts which were not immediately accessible to her. In this way the acquisition of language facilitated her building a model of her world.

A further example is an instance of fantasy play in which Suzanne uses language to reconstruct an episode which took place shortly beforehand. It illustrates how language can provide blind children with a powerful tool for understanding what is going on around them, and also serve as a medium for representing a distinction between 'self' and 'other'. Here Suzanne reproduces variations in tone of voice and discourse content to take up the positions of her mother, her sister and herself. In doing so she uses the pronouns *I* and *you*. Though she was not followed for long enough to plot the emergence of the *I/you* distinction in all its grammatical manifestations (this is not normally expected in sighted children before the middle of the third year, see E. Clark, 1978), this example and the one above indicate that she was already beginning to achieve what poses considerable problems for most blind children (Fraiberg, 1977).

Example 2.   Elaine is bouncing on and jumping off the settee. Suzanne (2;3) apparently appreciates something of what she is doing and in her own way attempts to copy her.
Suzanne: *'Laine, I'm* [laughing] *Whoops!* [she deliberately throws herself on the floor] *I fell over.*
The mother interferes and warns Elaine and then smacks her to discourage her exuberance. Shortly afterwards Suzanne laughs and apparently reconstructs the scene for herself.
Suzanne: *You's fall over!* [in her own voice]
Using a severe intonation, she then reproduces something of her mother's language.
Suzanne: *Now watch it! You asked this!*
The episode ends with a mock cry, presumably as a representation of Elaine, and further laughter from Suzanne.

Thus, by the close of the study, at two years three months, the early restrictions in Suzanne's language relative to sighted children had apparently

been resolved. She was naming and requesting objects frequently, referring to places beyond her range of touch, commenting on other people's possession of objects and on their actions where those actions where familiar to her. Though her mode of access to the environment and her sensory experience is different from sighted people's in crucial respects, the entry into language has given her a means both for extending her own awareness of what is going on around her and also for sharing in those events with other people. In a very real sense dialogue has provided a bridge to others, objects and the surrounding context, giving her a handle on the outside world.

CONCLUDING DISCUSSION

It is usually assumed that studying the development of children with such an apparently clearcut handicap as lack of vision will throw light on the processes involved in 'normal' development. The general method is to start with some theoretically based assumptions about the importance of vision or visually based systems to sighted children, using these assumptions to make more or less specific predictions about the likely consequences of blindness. Comparative studies are then undertaken with the aim of supporting or disconfirming the original theory. In practice, the original assumptions lead to the prediction of difficulties or delays for blind children. Since this is what is generally found, unfortunately the comparative studies rapidly reduce to demonstrations of the importance of what blind children lack, namely vision, to the children who have it, namely the sighted.

This chapter began in this tradition, by drawing predictions about the likely consequences of blindness for the emergence of language from recent work on sighted children. But particular limitations in such an approach may now be apparent. Apart from the fact that it tends to foster a totally negative view of blind children's development, or the assumption that they are like sighted children with 'something missing', such a framework can tell us little about what is involved in adapting to the difficulty. As a consequence practical implications must be speculated upon afterwards, rather than following directly from the research itself.

This might suggest that we should abandon the idea of using studies of handicapped groups to

enrich our understanding of the 'normal' process, and that comparative work can do little to help blind children themselves. One might argue that, if our primary concern is understanding how blind children acquire language, we should give priority to this population, concentrating on the uses which may be made of senses which they have rather than on those which they lack, and on the functions which language might serve for them. This could provide more adequate criteria for what constitutes developmental progress for blind children, and have implications for intervention as a direct outcome of the research itself. For example, one might use factors found to be associated with relatively satisfactory progress within the blind child population as the basis from which to design enrichment programmes.

However, in so far as blind and sighted children are growing up to speak 'the same language', some kinds of comparisons between the two populations are essential for clinical purposes, and it is, after all, only through processes of comparison that the notion of alternative routes in development can become tangible. But further than this, it is my contention that it is through examining alternative routes that the study of blind children can shed most light on the 'normal' process. This can be illustrated particularly clearly by looking at children whose development contradicts predictions drawn from the sighted child literature, as has been the case with Steven, Jerry and Suzanne. What does the relatively satisfactory development of these children do to the status of the original theories?

The issues raised by these three children's development are complex, less a question of simply proving the sighted child theories right or wrong than of revealing areas of inadequacy and inconsistency. For example, the close parallels between the development of these blind children and that of sighted children, in pre-verbal communication, the emergence of representation and broad features of language development, challenges any claim that lack of vision necessarily results in developmental delay. But this does not mean that vision is not important to sighted children. Rather it suggests that there is a problem in the way in which its role is usually conceived. Similarly, the notion of continuity between pre-verbal communication and early language is not disputed by these children's development. Indeed, the persistence of communicative procedures which were relatively idiosyncratic, or which are unlikely to be found as extensively in

fully sighted children, provides fairly strong support for continuity of function. But clearly the
relationship will have to be posed in a new way if
we are to account for how it is that blind children
discover functions for language, such as requesting
objects, which were not available in the pre-verbal
period. On the relation between cognitive development and language acquisition, the third major area
touched on in this chapter, these children's development is consistent with the notion that cognitive
change is integral to the emergence of language, as
has been argued for sighted children. However, the
gains in Suzanne's understanding which were made
possible, but not totally determined, by the entry
into language itself are not easily encompassed
within traditional approaches to the relation between language and thought. This suggests that a
new way of posing the relationship is necessary.

Understanding the alternative routes discovered
by these children does not, however, simply indicate
areas of inadequacy. In this case it has more specific implications for theoretical changes, or suggests areas where future research might be profitably directed. For instance, on the question of the
role of vision, the problem may lie in assuming that
any system has a necessary priority, functioning independently of others, as if they constitute separate faculties. Considering the three infants' interactions with their parents, for example, it was
true that the mother's use of alternative systems
led them to talk more and to use more physical contact than is typical of mothers interacting with
their sighted infants (see Urwin, 1978a). More
striking were the ways in which they used non-visual
systems simultaneously or interchangeably, and established correspondences across different sensory/
communication systems, as in the ways in which they
used their voices to match the babies' facial expressions, and mark body movement. Ultimately, it
is this potential for multiple access to and encoding of reality which makes it possible for children
lacking one kind of sensory experience to acquire
the language used by all. This suggests that further research should concentrate not on the senses
in isolation but on the relations between them and
on their potential substitutability. Though concerned with rather different questions, the work of
McGurk and MacDonald (1977) and Mills (Chapter 5)
on visual/auditory illusions and Landau's work
(Chapter 7) on the blind child's use of sighted
terms represent exciting examples in this direction.

Similar issues are raised by the question of how to account for the later emergence of language functions which are established pre-verbally through gesture in sighted children. Reflecting back on the sighted child literature, it now appears that the limitations may at least in part be due to a tendency to conflate form and function in development, and to disregard implications of actually acquiring words for changing the child's communication system. In the desire to demonstrate continuity, investigators have concentrated on the insertion of linguistic forms into pre-established communicative means, for example, on the use of indicating gestures followed by the use of indicating gestures plus standard words. These communicative acts are clearly related. But to assume that they are identical ignores the fact that the acquisition of words allows for a separation between form and function less available to the pre-verbal child, which may itself pre-empt further developments. What, for example, is the significance of the child's beginning to use the same word in a variety of communicative contexts, or different words to achieve similar ends? It may be that a closer examination of the diversification of the child's system may throw light on what 'lifts' the child out of pre-verbal communication into language proper. Furthermore, apart from providing a 'distance' from external reality, the insertion of words may change the nature of the child's interactions with other people dramatically. The implications of this were particularly marked in Suzanne's case, since it was through entering into verbal dialogue that she discovered new functions for language.

In attempting to argue for a relationship between language development and cognition, the sighted child work, discussed above, has relied on arguing for a correspondence between two-term semantic relations and underlying conceptual structures. Apart from the problem of accounting for the mapping mechanism which unites linguistic and cognitive structures (see Elliot, 1981), this argument is in accord with a more general tendency to assume that one is a reflection of the other, or that language and thought are in some way isomorphic. Yet language does not only map concepts or refer to things in the world. Meaning in language is also carried by connections or associations which operate between words themselves. That is, language allows for establishing connections across or between contexts, for marking relations of similarity, correspondence,

difference, and so on, a process which may itself bring into being new orders of meaning. It was through establishing such connections that Suzanne was led to understand what was unknown to her, as the mother used language to make the wider context accessible to the child by setting it in relation to what was already known.

Suzanne's development represents only one possible alternative route through which blind children can resolve early restrictions related to their limited access to the immediate context. Though using language to establish links across contexts is clearly particularly advantageous to blind children, it is important to recognize that the process described is not confined to blind children, or even only to children. It is, for example, integral to using language in teaching or explanation (Ortony, 1979). Walkerdine and Corran (1979), for example, have described strikingly similar procedures used by teachers helping children grasp mathematical concepts in a classroom situation. They have shown how the teacher begins with what is familiar to the child, and uses language to set up connections or correspondence across numerical groupings. This process both focusses the child's attention on the common underlying relation, and at the same time allows him or her to become aware of deficiencies or inadequacies in the previous assumption or explanation.

Such a viewpoint gives language, or rather the possibility which this creates for dialogue with others, a progressive role in the child's thinking. It is in marked contrast with the assumption underlying much of the earlier work on blind children's language carried out in educational establishments (e.g. Cutsforth, 1951). As I have argued elsewhere (Urwin, 1978b) the preoccupation with 'verbalism' and the lack of a framework for conceptualizing the advantages of language to blind children may have been major factors contributing to the paucity of work on how blind children actually acquire language. It is perhaps time to focus more attention on what blind children may gain through acquiring language, with respect to both their opportunities for social interaction and for their understanding of the wider environment. Further studies of parent-child discourse in the early stages would seem a useful point at which to begin.

Chapter 14.

THE INVESTIGATION OF VISION IN LANGUAGE DEVELOPMENT

Michael Garman

In the preceding chapter by Cathy Urwin we have a
balanced and careful consideration of early language
development in the blind child as seen in the context of some recent proposals on cognitive functioning in relation to language development in the
sighted child. It is a paper that invites some re-
flective discussion, I think, and I shall take up
three points for this treatment. First, though, I
have to make it clear that I am commenting as a linguist with a special interest in language development, including language disability in children, but
that I speak from no first-hand contact with the
language of the blind child.
    The first point concerns the possibility that
we might treat language acquisition by blind children as a testing ground - specifically, in this
case, for cognition-language relationships in early
language development. It is easy to see that specific predictions might be made about difficulties
in language acquisition by the blind child, given
what we currently think about the situation in the
sighted child; and the success of such predictions
in relation to the data might certainly be taken as
a useful test of our knowledge. To take a very
crude example: if reciprocal gaze between child and
adult is crucial to the establishment of (proto)con-
versational interchange (Bruner, 1975), and if conversational units are the building blocks of language acquisition (Dore, 1979), then we might expect
blind children to be at a disadvantage. Studies
like Urwin's suggest that we may indeed find some
disadvantages of blind children, but that there will
also be many overall similarities with sighted children. The important question for us, then, is, how
are such findings to be interpreted? When we find
specific and reliable difficulties, we can perhaps

conclude that they are indeed the result of blindness (although this statement may well be too simple). Faced with reliable similarities, on the other hand, we might conclude <u>either</u> that what we thought was crucial to language acquisition is not so crucial, after all, <u>or</u> that indeed it <u>is</u> crucial, but that blind children have compensated in some way. The upshot of the latter interpretation is that our prediction survives in spirit, even though it is apparently challenged. Following this up for a moment, it may lead us to consider a view of human language acquisition ability which says that, <u>given</u> intact vision, certain strategies will regularly be employed <u>en route</u> to certain language abilities, but also that <u>without</u> this faculty certain alternative (and ultimately specifiable) strategies are available, to achieve the same end. According to this view, it would be wrong to say that alternative strategies lead to 'deficient' language acquisition. It would also be wrong to say that our assumptions about the basic nature of sighted strategies are incorrect.

The second point leads on from this, since Urwin points out that 'developmental delay' may be a grossly misleading term for describing her subjects' performance. Speaking as a linguist who is concerned with language disability and with defining 'delay' versus 'deviance', and so on, I agree very strongly with the drift of this. Once the language system has started to develop, we must beware of over-interpreting certain gaps (e.g. lack of reference to objects out of touch) as evidence for 'language' disability. The relevant question is whether these gaps will eventually lead to language disability (see Elstner, Chapter 3). But first we must know what we want to call 'language disability'. Again, from a linguist's point of view, I would like to emphasize in this connection the following two requirements: (1) the need to distinguish difficulties in the use of language that arise from visual (or any other) handicap from the concept of specific linguistic disability. This might be expressed as communicative versus linguistic disability. The child's ability to implement successful referential acts (see Mulford, Chapter 9) is a case in point. This is certainly not to deny the reality or importance of communicative disability; it is simply to point out that, if linguists are to be involved in assessing blind children's language (a plea that has already, quite properly, been made by other contributors to this volume), we should try to understand

the fairly restricted area within which the linguist can be expected to make a professional contribution.

If we accept the distinction between communicative and linguistic disability, then how should we expect the linguist to approach the assessment of the blind child's language? This leads us to the second requirement: (2) establishing the relevant norms of assessment. Candidates, I think, are the following: (a) normal sighted language acquisition - the problem here being that we might expect typically to get what Urwin suggests, i.e. some differences but also some similarities with the blind child. This then brings problems of interpretation (as mentioned already) and a nagging sense that maybe we do not know as much as we thought we did about the sighted child with normal language. (b) The second possible norm is sighted language acquisition in the context of a specific linguistic disability - which might seem so obviously to compound our problems under (a) that it is not worth considering at all. But it is worth mentioning, I think, if only to underline the point that 'specific linguistic disability' is a neutral concept: i.e., where such disability exists (perhaps, say, in the form of some lexical semantic disability), linguists should be able to assess it, regardless of whether it occurs in a blind child, or a deaf child, or a child with mental handicap or with combinations of such handicaps - or, indeed, with no apparent cause for the disability at all. This is important, if the linguist's role is to make contact with intervention; the linguist's assessment must be independent of other (e.g. medical, psychological) terms of assessment, or it may contribute nothing that is new. It is also important in view of McGurk's reminder (McGurk, Chapter 10) that, as far as intervention is concerned, we ought to address ourselves to the problems of the vast majority of blind children, regardless of the fact that, for one reason or another, they may turn out to be unsuitably 'messy' subjects for the purposes of pure research. (c) The congenitally blind adult with normal language provides a third candidate norm, and this is worth considering because it may help us to understand more clearly how to separate out visual handicap from developmental factors; but this norm inevitably suggests a further one, (d) the sighted adult. This is in many ways our starting point. How do linguistically mature congenitally blind adults handle dialogue, for example, in a situation where there is ambiguity of reference, or indeterminacy of the

addressee's attention, simply by reason of visual
handicap? Do we want to deny congenitally blind
adults true linguistic maturity on these grounds? If
not, then the difference between the sighted and the
congenitally blind adult in such matters should not
be ignored when we assess the situation that blind
children find themselves in. Or, to put it another
way, once we have a clearer picture of the endpoint
of the blind child's linguistic development, we
stand a better chance of interpreting its midpoint,
and so on down. This approach should not <u>replace</u>,
but should arguably <u>complement</u>, the approach from
comparisons with the sighted child.

Thirdly, Urwin's study of Suzanne, carried on
into later stages of language development, clearly
suggests that aspects of linguistic development may
themselves serve as compensating elements in the
communicative system of the blind child. To quote
Urwin (I take this from her summary):

> The development of dialogue enabled [Suzanne]
> to discover new functions for language, such as
> requesting objects, and played a major role in
> extending her access to the surrounding con-
> text, including the activities and independent
> perspectives of other people.

So, whether or not language can be said to develop
via alternative strategies in the blind child, once
developed it may help to compensate for blindness.
It is perhaps because of this that we think of blind
adults as talking about the same world as sighted
adults, even though we know that some of their perceptions might be different. But this in turn
raises another comparison that might profitably be
studied, namely, the blind adult with normal language ability versus the blind adult with a specific
linguistic disability: the question to be asked
here is whether language is the only, or the best,
means of compensating for blindness.

Finally, I must acknowledge that I have defined
the linguist's role quite narrowly in what I have
said. I do so simply on the basis of my own experience and what I have learned (and this was a great
deal) from the other contributions to this volume.
Obviously, I am concerned to discover what should be
the appropriate role for the linguist in the assessment of the blind child's language. In what I have
outlined here there is, I believe, sufficient work
to be done! More importantly, working on lines such
as these, linguists might well be able to help

significantly with some (but surely not all) aspects of the language problems faced by young blind children.

Chapter 15.

LANGUAGE AND ACTIVE TOUCH: SOME ASPECTS OF READING
AND WRITING BY BLIND CHILDREN

Susanna Millar

The relation between language and active touch[1] is
arguably one of the most intriguing questions when
considering the development of the blind child.
Touch and movement, together with tone of voice,
provide much of the context necessary for acquiring
language. Without this context we expect 'verbalisms' and empty babble. Conversely, we also assume
that verbal strategies are particularly important
for the blind to mediate a number of other skills.
I believe these assumptions to be correct in the
main. Nevertheless, I shall argue here almost the
opposite case. I shall first present a finding
which suggests that even purely verbal associations
are not necessarily completely empty of meaning or
thought. Secondly, and this is my main argument, I
want to make the point that even in such language-
based skills as reading and writing, overly verbal
strategies can lead to spatial neglect and serious
inefficiency.

The Investigation of Semantic Incongruity
The finding which I want to present first provides a
corrective to our more usual preconception about
'verbalisms' in the blind. Clearly, totally congenitally blind children cannot know to what quality
colour names refer. It is, therefore, often assumed
that the use of colour terms by the blind must necessarily be merely empty and meaningless talk of the
kind that has come to be known as 'verbalism'. Of
course, blind children can and do learn appropriate
colour names for objects; but this could be due to
rote learning. It is not generally realized, however, that the congenitally totally blind, as I
shall show, can also make correct decisions about
inappropriate colour-object combinations which they

167

are very unlikely to have learned by rote.

Method

The experimental task which was presented to twelve
congenitally totally blind children was to judge
whether adjective-noun word pairs were appropriately
paired or not. The age range of the children was
eight to thirteen years, with a mean age of ten
years. Each of the blind children was paired with a
sighted child of the same age, sex, and socio-eco-
nomic status who had achieved the same verbal and
digit span scores as his blind cohort. The word
pairs were in four 'modality' blocks - auditory,
tactual, spatial and visual. All visual terms were
colour words. Half the pairs in each block were
appropriate adjective-noun combinations, such as
singing bird, hard wood, round ball and *red rose*;
the other half of the word pairs in each block were
inappropriate combinations, such as **barking cat,
*soft iron, *tall dwarf* and **black snow*. Appropriate and inappropriate pairs were interspersed randomly, and care was taken to balance the order of
blocks over subjects within each group. The subject's hands rested lightly on two response bars,
one designated for appropriate and one for inappropriate word pairs. These were also counter-bal-
anced. The instruction to the subject was to press
the relevant response bar as soon as possible when
hearing a word pair. Word pairs were spoken at
equal rates and a timer-counter was activated at the
beginning of each pair. Depressing the response bar
stopped the timer-counter so that latencies could be
recorded.

Results and Discussion

Overall, errors were negligible. Blind children had
an error rate of just under four per cent, and
sighted children's error rate was just under two per
cent. The youngest blind children did produce more
errors on visual and spatial adjectives, both with
inappropriate and appropriate pairs. This is hardly
surprising, since they will have had less opportunity to learn appropriate pairs. But the older blind
children made few errors of any kind. More importantly, error rates produced by the older blind
children were very low, even for the inappropriate
colour-noun pairs. This means that they were able
to come to correct decisions despite the fact that
they had never had experience of the relevant

perceptual quality.

The most interesting finding came from the analysis of latencies for correct responses (see Figure 15.1). This showed that the blind took significantly longer on inappropriate pairs than the sighted, but only in the visual modality, that is with inappropriate colour-noun combinations (p < 0.01). These decisions were also significantly slower than their own decisions on other word pairs, including appropriate colour-noun combinations (p < 0.01). This means not only that the blind were not responding by rote to the inappropriate colour-noun pairs, but that they must have thought about them longer. Clearly we need to know far more before we can be certain about the basis on which the blind make such judgments correctly. Presumably, inferences from appropriate pairs that they have learned and from what they know about other qualities that describe objects play a part in this.

Figure 15.1: Mean Latencies for Correct Responses by Blind and Sighted Children to Appropriate (A) and Inappropriate (I) Adjective-Noun Word Pairs Taken from Four Modalities of Perception

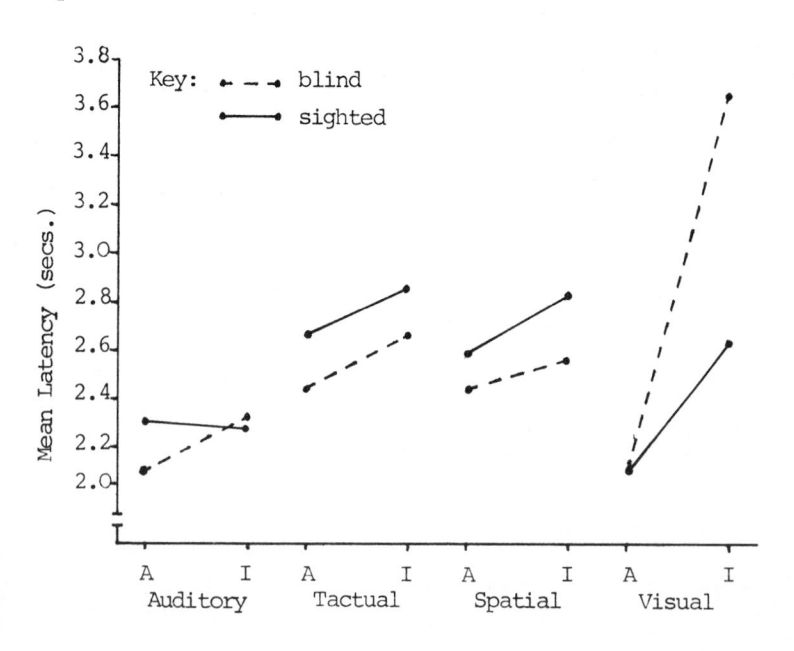

However, whatever the main basis of such decisions may be, the results allow us to reject the notion that purely verbal associations must necessarily be 'empty' in the sense that they are meaningless or cannot be thought about.

LANGUAGE AND BRAILLE READING

The main concern of this chapter is the use of language to mediate other skills, and particularly the fact that verbal strategies can lead to serious inefficiency when they involve a neglect of spatial coding. On the face of it, this seems to be something of a paradox, especially when applied to what is, after all, in the main a linguistic skill - namely reading. Spatial difficulties are rarely considered a problem in this, and there is indeed good evidence that the main difficulties of young sighted children fall in the linguistic field. Many recent formulations have stressed the importance of phonological analysis and coding (Frith, 1980). Deaf children who are very poor at this are typically also very retarded in reading (Conrad, 1979). It is also clear that blind children can remember more Braille letters when they are fast at naming them (Millar, 1975, 1978a). Nevertheless, purely verbal strategies can also have disadvantages in blind reading, and these need to be considered.

Models of Visual Reading
Most models of visual reading would present a picture of the processes involved which, in very simplified form, are graphically represented in Figure 15.2. Two main routes to reading, that is from the visual shapes on the page to the 'internal lexicon', are assumed: a visual route and a phonological route. The main argument has concerned the relationship between these two routes. On the one hand, it is argued that the visual string of letters on the page has to be translated first into sounds, or the phonological values associated with the letter shapes (Route B in Figure 15.2), before the meaning of the word can be accessed in a so-called 'internal lexicon'. On the other hand, it may be also possible to access the meaning in the 'lexicon' directly from the visual configuration (Route A in Figure 15.2) without translating it first into sounds by means of grapheme-phoneme correspondence rules (e.g. Coltheart et al., 1980).

170

Figure 15.2: Simplified General Visual Reading Model

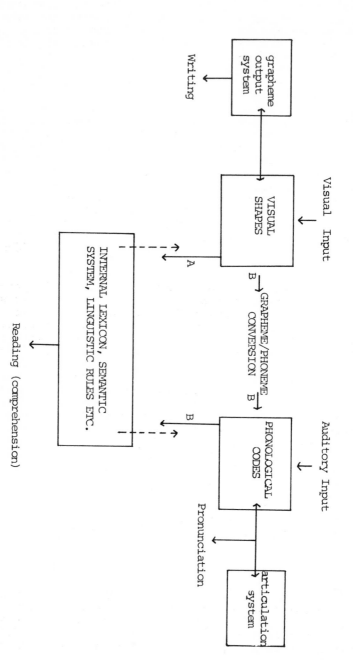

The semantic system also clearly affects the initial coding processes, as indicated by the broken lines in Figure 15.2. However, there seems to be little doubt when considering the visual route, whether it is conceived as direct or complex, that the reader codes the visual information on the page as shapes.

Models of Braille Reading

There are few explicit models of Braille reading. The main differences that are recognized between Braille and visual reading relate to the lack of redundancy in the Braille system, the use of contractions, the fact that it is necessary to read letter by letter rather than in global chunks, and that tactual recognition tends to be more difficult than visual recognition. The majority of the work done on Braille reading relates to the first three of these factors (Foulke, 1982). Clearly, both the lack of redundancy and the use of contractions impose extra burdens, including the learning of extra rules in addition to those necessary for visual reading. In the main, however, the difficulty of tactual recognition has received less attention. It is often blamed on poor tactual 'acuity' for which there is little remedy. Apkarian-Stielau and Loomis (1975) compare tactual perception to 'blurred' vision. Nolan and Kederis (1969) who did much to show up some of the major problems with the Braille system nevertheless assumed that Braille letters are coded as 'outline' shapes, much as they are indeed perceived in vision. However, the evidence that will be reviewed below suggests that the difficulty in the early stages of learning Braille is not due to poor tactual acuity, nor due to problems in associating the Braille letter shape with names, but rather to problems in recognizing the tactual dot patterns of Braille letters as global shapes or forms. In consequence, children sometimes get locked into verbal strategies, such as attempting to label the dots in a pattern by numbers, and failing to pay attention to the spatial relations between the dots in a pattern.

Experimental Findings on the Early Stages of Braille Reading: Non-spatial Coding of Raised Dot Patterns

There is evidence that tactual impressions can be coded in memory, and that such coding differs quite substantially from coding by name or verbal label (Millar, 1975). The paradigm used to demonstrate

this was adapted from Conrad (1971). The rationale
is that if children code items according to the
sound of the name, successive items in a list that
all have similar sounding names will be more difficult to remember than successive items which have
different sounding names. Similarily, if children
code letters according to the felt tactual impression, lists in which successive items are tactually
similar will be more difficult to remember than
lists in which successive letters are tactually dissimilar.

In order to establish, therefore, whether blind
children code letters by their verbal or by their
tactual characteristics, the children were tested on
lists of Braille letters that were either similar in
name-sound, or similar in feel, or dissimilar on
both counts. The difference between a subject's
scores on lists of similar and dissimilar sounding
Braille letters, and between scores on lists of letters with similar or dissimiliar tactual characteristics, showed whether they coded the letters by name
or by the tactual impressions. Both forms of coding
were found. Moreover, coding by name-sound was associated with an increase of the number of items remembered on the lists of dissimilar items. By contrast, tactual coding, shown by the difference between tactually similar and dissimilar lists, related to the number of remembered dissimilar letters in
precisely the opposite direction. Thus, tactual
coders remembered less; and the more a child relied
on coding by tactual impression rather than by verbal labels, the less he remembered. Nevertheless,
even children who relied on tactual coding alone
could remember up to three or four items. The
strategy is, therefore, not only possible but useful, although clearly different and inferior to verbal coding.

A similar result was found when blind children
were tested on Braille letters and raised-dot nonsense patterns (Millar, 1978a). Fast verbal recoding is an advantage. However, the results also
suggested that slow naming and a consequent reliance
on a relatively poor tactual code was not due to
verbal difficulties, but was rather due to the fact
that the tactual code is poorly organized. This
raised the possibility that the tactual impressions
that were remembered, were not, in fact, the physical shapes of patterns in the kind of global form
that are so easy to discern visually. Recent findings support this notion.

Braille letters are derived from a small, three

by two vertical by horizontal raised-dot matrix in which the presence or absence of any dot alters the pattern and consequently the letter for which it stands. Each letter of the alphabet also stands for a different word, and prefixes can alter their meaning still further. Not only the pattern of dots, but also their spatial position relative to one another, and relative also to a totally notional external frame, is of importance in determining what verbal label is to be applied to the character. Two dots at the top of the matrix, for example, do not mean the same when they occur at the bottom or in the middle. But while in sighted conditions the references to a top or bottom line for the matrix are visually clearly available, in blind conditions spatial reference presents considerable difficulties. In fact, the evidence from a number of different studies, and using different paradigms, suggests that children do not code the Braille patterns in terms of spatial parameters, let alone as global shapes, in the early stages of learning. The evidence has been surveyed in some detail elsewhere (Millar, 1981) and will consequently only be summarized here where relevant.

An important finding is the poor recall of tactual impressions of Braille letters under certain conditions. The notion, for instance, that tactual patterns are coded as global shapes, as they are indeed visually, would predict that generalization to enlarged size is easy. This is not so. Even when the letters are known in their normal format, and there is no difficulty in discriminating between the enlarged shapes, young Braille readers particularly have problems in recognizing those letters in enlarged format (Millar, 1977a). It has also been found that the number of dots in a shape is more important for discriminating it from another shape than differences in spatial features such as symmetry, or in the spatial relations between dots in a shape (Millar, 1978b). Precisely the opposite would be expected if the raised-dot patterns were coded as global tactual shapes.

On the assumption that Braille patterns are coded as shapes, it could also be expected that the left hand would always be superior in the early stages of reading, since the right hemisphere is involved in spatial perception, and information from the hands tends to go to the contralateral hemisphere (Milner, 1971). Reports on which is the 'better' hand for Braille reading tend, however, to vary with the number of years of Braille experience

the subjects have had (Fertsch, 1947; Millar, 1981).
Very early in learning there seems to be no hand
preference, even when discrimination accuracy is
quite good (Millar, 1977b).

The difficulty in coding small raised-dot patterns as global shapes by touch is not confined to
the blind, moreover. Blindfolded sighted ten-year-
olds were taught to name four Braille letters to a
reasonable criterion of accuracy. They were tested
on discrimination accuracy which was good; they were
then requested to draw the four letters they had
learned with the blindfold removed. It was clear
from the results that these bright ten-year-olds had
little idea of the spatial relations of dots in any
of the letters, and even less idea of the shape of
the letters (Millar, 1977b). The tactual impression
they relied on for naming varied between children,
but they clearly did not rely on the actual spatial
organization of the patterns. Naming the letters
seemed to have been based on some form of 'texture'
difference between the letters, which was related to
dot density rather than shape. In any case, the
difficulty of coding the patterns spatially does explain the rather poor performance with tactual codes
found earlier. It also suggests that difficulties
in learning the letters in the early stages of
Braille stem from a poorly organized spatial code
for the letters, rather than from difficulties in
naming as such. The apparent paradox that difficulties in the early stages of learning Braille may lie
with poor spatial coding, and an over-reliance on
verbal coding is strikingly illustrated by the case
of a congenitally blind girl who, at almost ten
years of age, was found to be completely unable to
read Braille.

The Case-Study of Helen
Helen, as she will be called here, was not merely a
case of severely retarded reading. The important
point is that, although she could not read, she
could write stories in Braille and her spelling was
as good as that of slightly younger but far more
intelligent girls. None of the usual explanations
therefore seemed to fit. Helen was a lively, talka-
tive but self-absorbed and rather babyish little
girl with an I.Q. in the region of low average on
the Williams test (Williams, 1956). However, this
low I.Q. clearly did not prevent her from learning
to write Braille letters, and indeed all the words
for which they stand, as well as many other

contractions and rules for their application.

Her learning, however, depended on producing the letters on the 'Perkins' key-board which is used for Braille writing in Britain. In the Braille matrix, the dots in the left column are numbered from one to three and those in the right column from four to six. Any letter can, therefore, be coded verbally by specifying the numbers of the dots it contains. Helen clearly associated the Braille dot numbers with the combination of fingers necessary to produce the letter on the 'Perkins' key-board. Her strategy in writing and spelling was instructive, and very easy to observe, since she called out all she did in a loud voice, without regard to those present, and even when requested not to do so. Any word to be written would first be spelled out by Helen aloud in terms of the dot-number combination of the letters, before she produced the combination on the Perkins Brailler. The strategy, which relied heavily on coding each dot in a letter verbally (by number) was perfectly adequate for writing. For reading it proved useless. Before a dot in a letter on the Braille page can be identified by number, its spatial position at least <u>vis-a-vis</u> the other dots must be recognized. This is precisely what Helen failed to do.

Helen had, of course, been known to be poor at reading for some time, but she had some very good strategies for disguising the extent of this deficit. Her fingers would travel expertly across the page while she recounted with few mistakes the story it contained. But she would still recount the story accurately even if the book were up-side down, or changed surreptitiously. She was clearly relying on memory. When she was first tested on letter naming, however, she showed an error rate of 69 per cent, and scored not a single three-letter word in one minute on test. At the same time, her letter discrimination was highly accurate. In contrast to the error rate at naming, her accuracy on discrimination tests was 77 per cent correct. This makes it necessary to reject the explanation, accepted previously, that Helen had especially poor tactual acuity.

The possibility that Helen might rely on coding 'texture' differences rather than on spatial coding of the shapes to a greater extent than other children was tested in a study which compared her with three other congenitally blind children. Two of the children (A and B in Figure 15.3) were approximately 18 months younger, but with intelligence quotients at a superior level; the third (C in Figure 15.3)

was a boy of the same age as Helen, with an average-
level I.Q. and reasonably fluent reading for his age.
A letter discrimination test was used with a ten-
second delay between the presentation of the standard and the test letter. To assess the main coding
strategy the children used, three types of interference tasks were interpolated in the ten-second delays. Verbal interference was tested by the repeti-
tion of *the..the..the* during delays, although verbal
coding was not expected as a basis for discrimination. Spatial interference was provided by having
the subjects repetitively feel around two shapes;
for texture interference subjects had to feel over
two textures during the delay. Figure 15.3 shows
the proportion of errors with the different types of
interference during delays. It is clear that Helen
showed over twice the proportion of errors with texture interference than with shapes, although these
also involved feeling across surfaces.

Figure 15.3: The Proportions of Errors for Helen and Blind
Subjects A, B and C on Successive Letter Matching with Verbal,
Spatial and Texture Interferences.

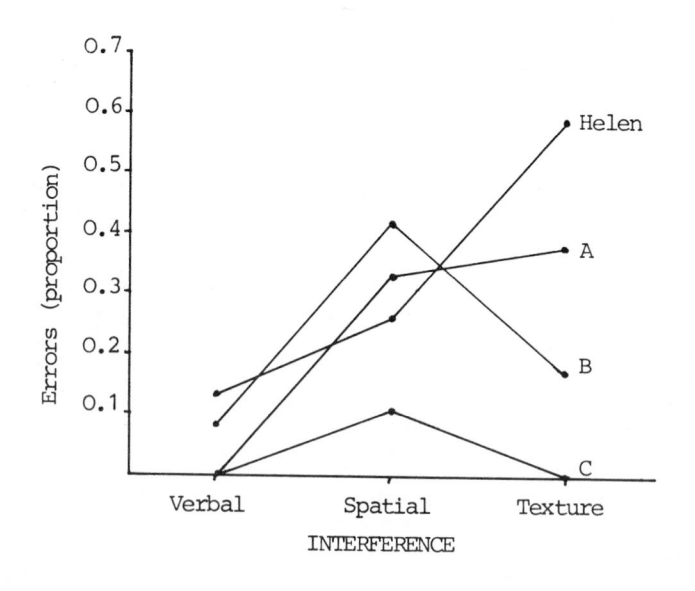

On verbal tests Helen did not differ from the others. For instance, she scored as well on producing and recognizing rhymes as the other three rather more intelligent children. She was well-known for her good verbal memory which, as mentioned above, enabled her to pretend to read. She had also long been known to be poor at spatial tasks, although even here some of her verbally-cued strategies helped her to disguise this at times. More importantly, her retardation in reading had been considered a symptom of poor tactual acuity and general backwardness rather than one of the results of her spatial difficulties. On test, she was found not to have the slightest idea that the Braille dots on the page lined up vertically on each side, and she required a great deal of intensive training before she was able to connect the relative spatial position of the dots with the number labels she was able to employ in spelling and writing. With spatial training she achieved an accuracy of 69 per cent on letter naming after six weeks. It took a further seven months before she achieved any reading age at all on a word speed test. However, her training had to include how to find the left side of her book in order to start reading, despite the fact that she had clearly been taught a very good means of doing so by first finding the spine of the book and working outwards from there. Thus, she was able to say from the outset that the spine of a closed book should be on the left. For Helen, the 'left' meant the side that her left hand was touching.

Verbal versus Spatial Coding

Helen's rather extreme case of dissociation between reading and writing must be explained at least in part by the discrepancy between her spatial and verbal skills, leading to an almost total neglect of spatial coding. The difficulty in teaching her was not so much that she could not learn spatial strategies, but that, left to herself, she would forget to use them and revert to the verbal means which for her were easier. In fact, Helen's case and the findings mentioned earlier, namely that it is difficult to code small tactual dot patterns in terms of spatial references or global form, make very good sense when the conditions of blind exploration are considered. Firstly, when exploring blind, there are no external references to which the dot patterns or the dots in a pattern can be referred. Secondly, the patterns are too small for it to be possible to

use self-referent anchors. Thirdly, unless the shape is already known, exploring movements tend to be too rapid and unsystematic to preserve anchor information. When I first started work in this field, I was rather scandalized one day to hear a good Braille teacher admonish a child for moving or rubbing his finger over a letter. He should keep his finger still. Evidently, she had found this useful advice, although it went against all we apparently know about the superiority of active over passive touch. The puzzle is clearer now: the top and sides of a relatively passive finger can provide a spatial frame to which dot positions in a letter can be referred. Fast naming must become easier in that case.

The evidence reviewed so far suggests that difficulties in spatial coding are almost inherent in the tactual perception of dot patterns. Indeed, it now seems rather doubtful that even non-retarded readers code the patterns as outline shapes. The evidence comes from twelve blind children, six of whom could be regarded as retarded readers since their word reading age lagged some two years behind their mental age. They had a mean chronological age of 10;3 years; a mean I.Q. of 101 (Williams test), and a mean word reading age of 8 years. The other six children had a chronological age of 10;1 years, and a mean I.Q. score of 97, while their mean word reading age was 9;11 years and thus commensurate with the level that would be expected at that age. It was argued that if non-retarded readers used outline-shape coding more than retarded readers, it would be expected that presenting the initial letter as an outline shape should speed recognition of shape identity of a second letter. Moreover, presenting the second or test letter as an outline shape should also be better if subjects code the initial letter in terms of its outline shape. However as Figure 15.4 shows quite clearly, errors for both retarded and non-retarded readers were higher in both conditions in which the letter was presented as an outline shape than for matching letters in their normal format. The difference was highly significant ($p < 0.001$) in an analysis of variance with the appropriate factors. Matching by dot patterns was also faster, for both the retarded and non-retarded readers, than matching dot patterns with outline shapes, although there was some indication in the latency data that for the non-retarded readers cuing by outline shape was faster than cuing by dot pattern. The effect was shown by a significant

interaction (p < 0.05) between retarded versus non-retarded readers and the letter type that had been presented. However, the relation was by no means as large as would be expected according to the hypothesis that the better readers habitually code Braille characters by their outline shape. A much slower process than form recognition seems to underly the recognition of the tactual impression from the page. There is good evidence already (Foulke, 1982) that tactual reading, unlike visual reading, tends to proceed far more as a letter-by-letter sequential process. But the evidence reviewed here suggests that even the letter, as a perceptual form, is not the unit of tactual reading. It is perhaps somewhat surprising that this was the case, even for the non-retarded readers in the above experiment whose ability to name and read words was not in question.

Figure 15.4: The Proportion of Errors and Latencies for Correct Responses in Retarded and Non-retarded Braille Readers in Successive Matching of Braille Letters according to Format.

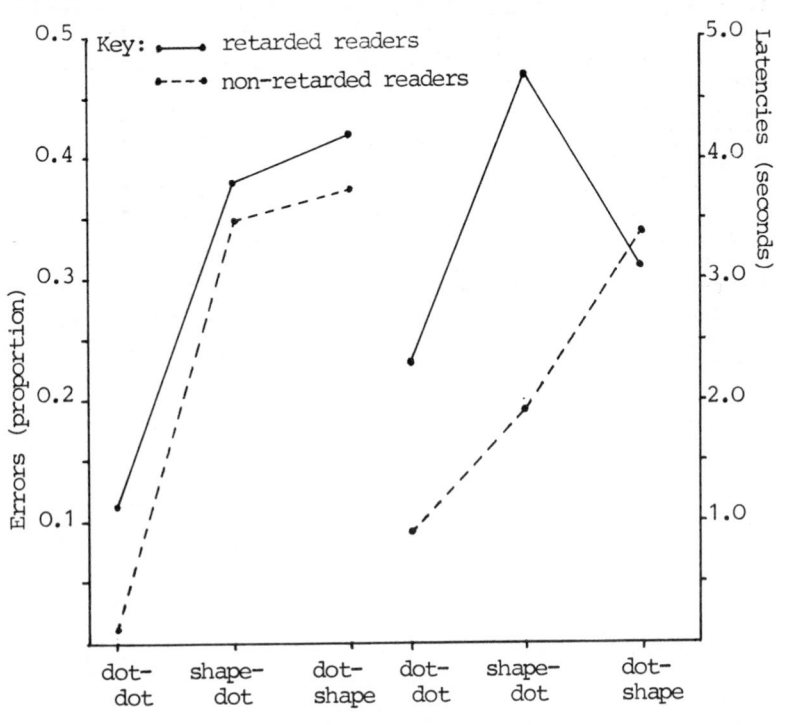

But this finding suggests that there is access to naming and meaning from tactual impressions that are not coded as global shapes. This process itself is not yet well understood.

One further point needs to be made in comparing the use of verbal strategies in tactual versus visual reading. Visual reading and writing provide feedback for each other. Thus visual writing uses movements that follow the same shape as the visually perceived character on the page. Braille writing, on the other hand, is not based on the shape of the Braille letter. On the contrary, it depends on depressing a combination of keys that, at least on the Perkins Brailler used in Great Britain, are arranged horizontally on the keyboard. The Braille letter on the page based on the three by two matrix, on the other hand, has a vertical organization. If Braille readers were to use spatial information to relate reading and writing, therefore, they would have to perform a 90 degree mental rotation, in the opposite direction for the two hands. It seems extremely unlikely that young blind readers can do this, the more so as young blind children tend to have particular difficulties with mental spatial rotation tasks. To relate reading and writing, therefore, the Braille reader, at least at the outset of reading, is again forced to use a verbal mediating strategy. The more obvious strategy, used by most blind children at the outset, is to label the keys on the Brailler with the appropriate dot number. The keys which are depressed by the fore-, middle- and ring-fingers of the left hand are labelled with the numbers one to three, since these produce the left-hand column of dots in a letter; the keys depressed by the corresponding fingers on the right hand are labelled from four to six, since these produce the right-hand column of a Braille letter. Clearly without some means of coding the dots on the page spatially, the dots cannot be identified even by number. But the temptation to rely on verbal strategies as much as possible at the expense of spatial coding, even when that is needed, must be very great.

The Implications for a Model of Braille Reading
The evidence reviewed here on the very early stages of Braille reading suggests that, even in its simplest form, any Braille reading model would have to postulate rather more stages or connections than seem to be absolutely necessary for visual reading.

Whereas, in visual reading, we can accept that even the beginning reader will perceive a string of shapes on the page, this is clearly not possible for Braille. Memory for tactual impressions exists. Evidence from a number of different studies, using converging methods, shows that in the initial stage of reading these tactual impressions are not necessarily organized spatially, let alone as global shapes. Such non-spatial tactual coding, possibly in terms of rather crude 'texture' differences, seems to occur particularly when naming or fast verbal recoding is difficult. But tactual coding does not depend on difficulties in verbal coding. In matching tasks, for instance, tactual coding may be faster (Millar, 1977a) and, therefore, more useful.

Tactual impressions can be associated with names to a limited extent. It was found, for instance, that sighted children could name four Braille letters which they could not draw as shapes (Millar, 1977b). Even when first tested, Helen was able to name some letters, although very few, and not very reliably. Thus, a model must allow for the possibility of connections between the non-spatial tactual impression on the page and naming or meaning. On the other hand, as the evidence from Helen shows, such non-spatial tactual codes are obviously not sufficient for learning to name all the Braille letters, punctuation signs and contractions. Without some spatial analysis of the dots on the page and their relation to each other, it would be impossible even to keep the finger travelling along the letter string without moving to a different line. For letter recognition and word naming, an analysis of the relative spatial position of dots is in fact essential. However, from the evidence of the middle-school-age readers discussed earlier, it seems clear that, even for the non-retarded readers, the unit of reading is not the global letter shape.

Figure 15.5 is an attempt to represent some of the complexity of routes that seem to operate at least at the early stages of reading. Routes labelled A in Figure 15.5 represent the direct route and Routes B the indirect route (via the phonological system) between the shapes on the page and the internal lexicon.

On the basis of the evidence, our - very tentative - Braille reading model needs at least two more types of connection between the tactual impressions on the page and the naming, rule and lexical systems.

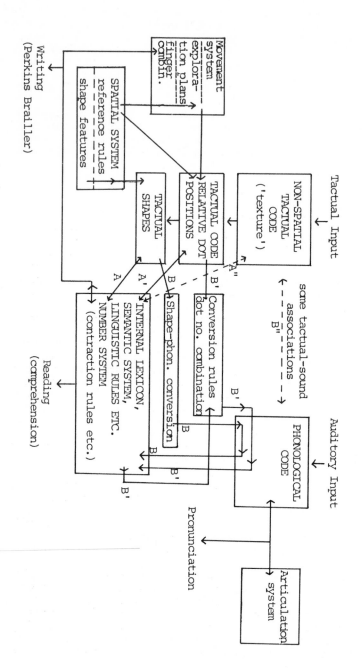

Figure 15.5: Simplified Tactual Braille Reading Model

One type of connection must run from the non-spatially coded impression (Routes A" and B" in Figure
15.5) and is here represented by a broken line to
show that these have limitations. Another type of
connection (Routes A' and B' in Figure 15.5) must be
via a code that makes use of some form of spatial
analysis of the relations of the dots to each other
which is at least sufficient to label each dot in a
letter pattern with its number in a matrix. The
model also shows that the tactual codes require some
input from the spatial system. A dot-numbering system in association with finger combinations is also
needed. Most paths are shown as effective in both
directions. Indeed, top-down processing in which
higher order meaning and context are used is probably more important for Braille than for visual reading.

Presumably, at a somewhat more advanced level
of reading when letters or words even may be processed as whole shapes, yet a third connection is
needed. As yet relatively little is known about the
means of achieving fast and fluent reading in
Braille (Foulke, 1982). The point here is that even
letter-by-letter sequential processing does not account for the reading process in non-retarded middle
school children. For these children the unit of
reading seems to depend on a still slower sequential
process of identifying the relative spatial positions of each dot and gap within patterns. Many
children, other than Helen, interpose a verbal system between the dot pattern on the page and reading
for either sound or meaning at this point, namely
that of naming the dots in terms of their position
number in the Braille matrix. This cannot be done
without identifying their relative spatial position,
however, which is precisely the point at which Helen
failed.

A question that must be asked in connection
with this model is whether all these possible routes
are obligatory. We do not as yet have an answer to
this. The dot numbering system, for instance, may
help precisely because the dot positions, although
coded spatially, are not organized as spatial wholes
or shapes at that point in learning. The numbering
system would make it easier to remember the dot combinations not in terms of position, but as digit
combinations that can be held in "working memory"
(Baddeley, 1976) so that their integration into
words and sentences becomes possible. Certainly, if
the connection with writing is to be established, a
common numbering system between the three by two

upright matrix on the page and the horizontally arranged key-board may be important. Interposed also
between the dots as tactual impressions on the page
and the meaning they bear for the child as letters
or words, or contracted parts of words, are quite
explicit rules that the Braille reader must learn
and master before he can 'perceive' a given pattern
correctly. These rules are indeed 'obligatory' for
reading beyond the first grade of Braille. However, no child would ever become a fluent Braille
reader if all the routes were obligatory. Many of
them presumably become so automatic that they drop
out with practice. Not all the routes are needed
either, for example for comprehension, for appreci-
ating poetry sounds, or for detecting a false tactual pattern in proof-reading. The fact is, however,
that fast Braille reading is difficult to achieve.
There seem to be two reasons for this: the difficulty of coding small raised-dot patterns in terms
of spatial parameters, and the need to incorporate
verbal rules and strategies, with a consequent tendency to rely too much on such strategies.

SUMMARY

The main argument in this chapter has been that our
preconceptions about the relation between language
and active touch in the blind child's thinking and
performance can lead us seriously astray. Prima
facie, it seems obvious that one of the greatest obstacles to the blind child's comprehension of written as well as spoken language is to have categories
of empty concepts, that is words and descriptions
which are without meaning because it is impossible
that the child should have experienced the referents
by touch or by any other remaining sense. Colour
words are the most extreme example of this, and so
constitute a test case. The fact that the congenitally totally blind can make correct inferences even
in understanding these shows that their so-called
'verbalisms' are not as empty as we normally assume.
It suggests also that the main obstacle to comprehension does not lie in the absence of experienced
qualities.
    Almost the converse case was argued about our
intuitions on the role of language in mediating other skills, and our assumptions about the information
necessarily provided by touch. The advantages of
fast verbal recoding for memory, and of verbal
strategies in relating Braille reading and writing,

for instance, are obvious enough. But, as Helen's extreme dissociation of reading and writing showed, an over-reliance on verbal mediating strategies can become a serious hindrance when it leads to a neglect of the information provided by touch, and particularly to a neglect of the spatial coding of this information. Such a neglect is often difficult to recognize, because we assume that patterns are coded by touch as they are in vision, that is that our finger feels the simple outline shape of a tactual dot pattern in the same way as we can see it on the page. The main problem for reading would then reduce to the difficulty of associating the name or sound with that pattern, with or without conversion rules. However, the fact that we <u>can</u> perceive shape by touch does not necessarily mean that this is what we do feel. On the contrary, the studies reviewed here showed that it is extremely difficult to feel the small raised-dot patterns of which Braille consists as outline shapes. It was shown that they are not even felt as such by children who can read Braille quite well, and that there is an even earlier stage in reading where the tactual impression coded in memory depends on such factors as dot density rather than on the spatial relation between the dots. The findings suggest that there are relationships between the naming and semantic systems and all three forms of tactual coding, although these may differ according to whether tactual impressions are encoded non-spatially, or organized at least in terms of dot position, or when they are involved in fluent reading. In comparison with visual reading, the influence of the naming and of semantic systems thus seems to be more complex and pervasive at all stages of learning to read by touch. Moreover, the very verbal strategies that children may use to compensate for the difficulty of coding the dot patterns spatially can become a hindrance to tactual reading.

NOTES

1. My research work described in this chapter was undertaken with a grant from the Social Science Research Council of Great Britain.

Chapter 16.

THE IMPLICATIONS OF RESEARCH FINDINGS ON BLIND
CHILDREN FOR SEMANTIC THEORIES AND FOR INTERVENTION
PROGRAMMES

Richard F. Cromer

The mark of a good paper is that it stimulates
thoughts in directions that are perhaps rather different from those of immediate concern to the author. The presentation by Susanna Millar in the
previous chapter gives us not only a review of her
carefully designed experiments on Braille reading by
blind children but also an intriguing case history
in the great tradition of neurology and neuropsychology. This potent combination provokes a number
of thoughts on a variety of related issues, and in
this discussion I will focus primarily on two: (1)
the need for clearly distinguishing and relating the
two different domains of conceptual thought and semantic encoding, and (2) problems that must be considered by those directly concerned with intervention procedures - in this case the teaching of
Braille to blind children.

DISTINGUISHING CONCEPTS AND SEMANTICS

Millar's first experimental finding, that blind
children are significantly slower on making decisions on incongruous adjective-noun colour-object
pairs while nevertheless giving correct replies,
clearly demonstrates semantic processing by these
children. These colour terms, she claims, are not
"empty verbalims" as some of the language of the
blind has been occasionally described in the past,
but are terms which are actively thought about and
responded to. In an earlier chapter, Barbara Landau
has already demonstrated that visual terms such as
look and *see* are not semantically empty. That the
terms the blind use might in the past have been
thought to be empty verbalisms comes from a lack of
differentiation of concepts and semantics (see

Werth, Chapter 8). Many psychologists have used these words as if they were interchangeable, but there is now increasing realization of the need to distinguish clearly between them.

Katherine Nelson (1978) has criticized most models of so-called "semantic memory" for the failure to differentiate between real world knowledge and word meaning. She defines the conceptual level as being what the child learns about the world. By contrast, the semantic level includes both the lexical level (the meaning of words) and knowledge of the relations among words and word meanings. Nelson suggests that in development the lexical level is built up independently of the conceptual level, and that the child must find ways of making appropriate connections between the two. Similarly, Susan Carey (1978) clearly distinguishes what she calls the child's conceptual domain and his lexical or semantic domain. The conceptual domain is the mental representation by which the world is understood. By contrast, the lexical domain is the structured set of words that encodes aspects of the conceptual domain. Each domain has its own identity and structure. This differentiation has often been muddled by psychologists (for example, in the confusion of "semantic memory" with "conceptual memory"), but it is basic in linguistics and anthropology. Sperber (1975), for example, has expressed this distinction by pointing out that semantic knowledge is about categories and not about the world. He considers the sentence *The lion is an animal*, and points out that to know the lion is an animal is not to know anything about lions, not even that they exist, as is shown by the sentence *The unicorn is an animal*. The English speaker knows the sentence *A spinster is an unmarried woman* to be true even if he knows nothing about matrimonial law. As Sperber (1975, p. 91) puts it:

> We might conceive of a machine capable of correctly indicating all the paraphrases, analytic tautologies and contradictions, in short, a machine that would possess all the semantic knowledge on which a language is based, without having, for all that, the least knowledge of the world.

Real world knowledge is termed "encyclopaedic knowledge" by Sperber. Statements of real world knowledge, e.g., *The unicorn does not exist*, are true or false according to the state of the world, and no

semantic rules determine their truth value.

During childhood, each domain can develop separately before the mapping of one domain onto the other occurs. Carey (1978) notes, for example, that pre-verbal infants and animals have knowledge of the domain of colour, as can be demonstrated in tests of perceptual matching, in the absence of any corresponding lexical or semantic encoding. This has also been demonstrated for groups who speak languages that only encode limited portions of the colour spectrum. Rosch (1977) has demonstrated that the Dani of Indonesian New Guinea perceive the same focal colours as other human groups even though their language has only two colour terms, *mili* and *mola*.

Since the conceptual and semantic domains are separate, there can at the same time be development within the lexical domain. Thus, the child can be acquiring colour words and semantic knowledge about their use as category words even though he is unable to map these terms correctly onto perceived colour differences. Elsa Bartlett (1978), in a carefully designed study of colour word acquisition in children, found that the children who were the least advanced at naming colours typically produced three or four colour terms without using any of the terms correctly. Young children can often list the names of several colours in response to questions such as *Do you know any colours?* before they know how to map those terms correctly onto the perceptual/conceptual domain. This may help to clarify some aspects of language in the blind. Blind individuals know a great deal about the structure of the lexical domain of colour without ever mapping it onto perceived colours.

The separation of conceptual knowledge from verbal or semantic knowledge has also been demonstrated in cases of brain pathology. For example, Marie-France Beauvois (1981) reports experiments on patients suffering from optic aphasia who will give the wrong name for an object, but correctly mime its use. Shown a picture of a boot, they will correctly pantomime the pulling on of the boot while misnaming the object completely. It would appear that conceptual meaning can be encoded motorically and by images; conceptual meanings exist independently of the semantics of the verbal system and can be encoded by other means.

The important distinction between conceptual and semantic knowledge is implicit in Vygotsky's claim (1962) that language and thought have

different roots. Slobin (1978) is studying the language development in children in widely differing
language groups in order to explicate the relationship between linguistic and conceptual knowledge in
development. One important task for the child is to
figure out just which aspects of a particular conceptual notion are encoded in the language of his
community.

It is interesting that blind individuals acquire some semantic knowledge before or without conceptual knowledge. It has already been argued that
young sighted children do this with colour words,
but the process may be highlighted in blind children. What Susanna Millar's experiment so nicely
demonstrates is that the language acquired by the
blind is not "empty". The words and phrases they
use are not learned by rote, but represent meanings
and categories that are actively manipulated and
thought about. This was particularly clearly demonstrated when it was shown that colour words, for
which the blind have no perceptual mappings, were
nevertheless responded to correctly in their semantic pairings, and with reaction times indicating active thought processes.

INTERVENTION PROCEDURES AND BRAILLE READING

The main claim of Millar's paper concerns the nature
of coding in the reading of Braille. Millar presents evidence that young Braille readers initially
use a non-spatial texture coding in which the density of the dots is taken as the crucial differentiating factor for letter identification. She claims
that shape coding is superior but that there is little evidence of its use by beginning readers of
Braille; Millar therefore suggests the need for directing attention to spatial coding skills instead of
relying on verbal strategies, especially in the early stages of teaching Braille reading. The implication for intervention techniques in the teaching of
Braille is that shape coding should be actively
taught and encouraged. It is worthwhile, therefore,
to consider some of the issues that may be of importance in considering intervention procedures with
any handicapped group, and to see in what ways these
issues specifically affect suggestions for the
teaching of Braille reading.

The first consideration concerns whether an observed deficiency is due to a real deficit or whether it is due to an elective strategy of avoiding

a non-salient system. Specifically, do the blind
suffer from a spatial deficit as a result of their
blindness, or do they merely avoid spatial encoding
due perhaps to its lessened salience because of the
lack of visual input? One way to consider this issue is by analogy to another handicapped group, the
deaf. O'Connor and Hermelin have conducted a number
of experiments on the ability of deaf children to
deal with temporally ordered phenomena. One experimental procedure (Hermelin and O'Connor, 1973) consisted of the presentation of short strings of numbers in a manner that was compatible with either
spatial or with temporal encoding. The apparatus
consisted of three small windows arranged horizontally. Below these was a single, fourth window. In
one condition, three numbers appeared in the upper
windows one after the other - one number in each
window. These numbers appeared in such a way, however, that they did not occur in a left-to-right order. For example, take the numbers 3, 9, 7 presented one after the other (temporally). These might be
presented such that the 7 occurred in the left-hand
window, the 3 in the central window, and the 9 in
the right-hand window. Thus, spatially, the left-
to-right presentation would be 7-3-9, whereas temporally, first-to-last, the numbers would have appeared 3-9-7. After a one-second interval the numbers were exposed one after another in the single
window below. This recognition display could show
the numbers as they had appeared in temporal order
(3-9-7), spatial order (9-7-3) or else randomly
(e.g. 9-7-3). The child's task was to judge whether
the order of the two presentations was the same or
different. The task was the same for a second, similar condition in which the initial presentation was
successive, in the lower window, and the recognition
task was based on the subsequent three-window display. This three-window display was presented either temporally congruent, spatially congruent, or
randomly. Hermelin and O'Connor found that hearing
children generally gave temporally ordered recognition responses. Only 3 out of 40 children (7.5 per
cent) recognized the left-to-right but not the
first-to-last order of the digits. By contrast, 31
out of 57 deaf children (54.5 per cent) recognized
the spatially ordered display but not the temporally
ordered one. Thus, even when the element of spatial
display was eliminated by the use of a single window
either for the recognition display or in the second
condition for the initial input, more than half of
the deaf children failed to recognize the previously

presented temporal sequence. These results appear to confirm other findings that deaf children have difficulties with temporally ordered information. However, O'Connor and Hermelin (1973a,b) went on to carry out further experiments that showed that the deaf children were not unable to process temporally ordered information; rather, they use spatial information where they can as a preferred strategy. For example, in one of these experiments (O'Connor and Hermelin, 1973a), 20 hearing and 20 congenitally deaf children viewed material such as photographs of faces presented in five windows. As in the other experiments, the temporal, first-to-last order of the items was incongruent with the spatial, left-to-right order. In another condition 40 deaf and 40 hearing children saw similar items presented successively at the same location. The child's task was the same for both conditions: after viewing the material, the child was shown two temporally adjacent members of the set of five, and he had to tell the experimenter which one had come first. Thus, in this experiment, the children were required to retain only temporal order information. Under these conditions no differences were found between the hearing and deaf children. In other words, when the deaf are instructed to retain only temporally ordered information, they are as efficient as hearing children. This shows that in other experiments, like those mentioned previously, where spatial information is available, the deaf evidence an elective strategy to utilize such information; but they do not have an incapacity to appreciate temporal order.

What about the blind child's use of texture coding rather than spatial coding in the reading of Braille? Millar has presented evidence that Braille dot patterns are not coded as outline shapes. A more comprehensive review of her findings can be found in Millar (1978b). She has shown that better Braille readers make a greater use of spatial coding than the poorer readers, but even here the differences were not as great as would be expected. In any case, it would appear that nothing prevents a blind individual from making use of spatial coding of the Braille letters; rather, he is unlikely to do so unless given special instruction - and, if I understand Millar's position correctly, this is what she is advocating. Further evidence that the blind are not impaired in using spatial coding comes from some findings which are in conflict with those reported by Millar. Millar reasons that since the

right hemisphere is responsible for spatial perception, a left-hand advantage for Braille reading should be found if the early learner is coding the material spatially. Her experiments (Millar, 1977a) show no left-hand advantage early in learning. However Hermelin and O'Connor (1971a,b) have reported left-hand superiority for Braille readings not only in adults, but in children. However this discrepancy of results on blind children is eventually resolved, there is evidence of left-hand superiority in adult Braille readers, indicating that spatial encoding is possible, and thus the thrust of Millar's argument – that spatial encoding may need to be actively encouraged – is well taken. It would appear that, in the blind, nothing prevents spatial coding, and therefore one could presumably strengthen its use.

This brings us to a second issue in intervention: is it better to use intervention strategies to strengthen weak or little-used skills, or instead to direct effort to building up compensatory skills? Millar implies that spatial coding is necessary for good Braille reading. Yet she found that even good readers of Braille made significantly more errors in conditions in which letters were presented as outline shapes, indicating continuing use of texture codes. Furthermore, even if younger or poorer Braille readers make greater use of texture coding, they are nevertheless reading, albeit by a non-optimal method. There is some evidence that blind children prefer to use tactual cues rather than spatial ones in cognitive tasks unrelated to Braille reading (see e.g. Cromer, 1973). It would appear that Braille reading can occur whichever type of coding is primarily used. In designing intervention programmes, consideration must therefore be given to the best method which will engage the child in mastering the task. Again, analogies to other fields may be useful. Here, we can consider the kinds of issues raised by research on reading skills and the application of various intervention procedures to dyslexic children.

Studies of adult aphasic patients with acquired reading difficulties have provided some insight into the processes that can be used in that skill. Marshall and Newcombe (1973, 1977) were able to classify patients into groups in terms of which of two basic methods they used on a task requiring them to read single words without context. One method uses a phonemic route in which a word is converted into a sound before it is interpreted. The other

method employs a direct semantic route in which the meaning of a word is recovered directly from its visual appearance. The advantage of the phonemic route is that it allows for the pronunciation and reading of new, unfamiliar words. It would thus appear that reading instruction for normal children or intervention programmes with dyslexic children should encourage phonemic coding strategies. The issue is, however, more complex than these findings imply.

Snowling (1980) studied a group of 18 dyslexic children of mean chronological age 12;1 who were substantially behind their peers in reading ability. In this group, the low reading scores could not be attributed to low intelligence, the mean I.Q. being 106. The children in this group were compared to 36 normal readers who were matched in terms of reading age. The task was to make same/different judgments for pronounceable nonsense words presented either auditorially or visually. The four conditions consisted of auditory or visual presentation of the first word coupled with either auditory or visual presentation of the word to be judged as same or different from the first. Both groups did well on the auditory-auditory task. This shows that the dyslexic children had no problems with auditory discrimination. However, there was a significant difference on the visual-auditory task - the task that is most similar to normal reading - with the dyslexic group scoring poorly. Since the groups were matched in terms of reading age, Snowling concluded that the dyslexic readers perform in a qualitatively different manner from normal readers. These dyslexic children evidence a specific impairment in grapheme-phoneme translation; they are not just the low end of a normal distribution of readers.

Jorm (1979) has reviewed evidence on dyslexic children that leads to the same conclusion that these children have difficulty with a phonological route to meaning. He attempts to explain this in terms of a short-term memory deficit. Whatever the true reason for their grapheme-phoneme impairment, suggestions for remediation programmes become apparent. Jorm argues, for example, that because dyslexics can access words visually but have difficulties in using the phonological route, methods of instruction should capitalize on their intact system. Thus, he suggests that the look-say method may be more effective for this group of children than phonic methods that try to teach grapheme-phoneme correspondences. Nevertheless, the great value of

the phonemic method is that it allows the reader to
access the meaning of unfamiliar and novel words -
and this leaves the interventionist with a dilemma:
does one use methods of instruction that are directed to the strengths of the individual, as Jorm seems
to suggest, or does one use methods addressed to improving a poorly functioning system in that individual, but a system that has overall advantages for
him? The best method of instruction may depend on
the type and degree of impairment.

Frith (1981), in a review of work on dyslexia,
suggests that the kind of intervention programme
should depend on the specific handicap in the child.
She reviews evidence that dyslexia is a specific
deficit and that dyslexic children are not just poor
readers at the low end of a scale of reading ability. That is, specific reading deficit (dyslexia)
can be distinguished from general reading retardation. Frith cites the epidemiological studies of
Rutter and his colleagues (1970, 1975, 1976) who
show that this distinction is supported by three
kinds of evidence. The first is statistical.
Rutter and Yule (1975) point out that there is a
hump at the lower end of the normal curve of distribution of reading scores. This hump is accounted
for by children with specific reading deficits. The
second type of evidence is aetiological. The specific and general groups differ in terms of a number
of psychological, neurological and social factors.
In particular, the children with specific reading
deficits show stronger associations with speech and
language delays. The third type of evidence - educational - is the most important in terms of the
current claim. It has been found in a follow-up
study after four to five years that the effectiveness of remedial teaching is greater for the group
with general reading retardation than for the group
with specific reading deficit. Frith points out
that it is this persistence over time and the relative lack of response to conventional teaching methods that most effectively distinguishes specific
reading deficit from general reading retardation.
This has important educational implications. As
Frith (1981, p. 99) has put it:

> ...it might well turn out that a dyslexic child
> benefits more from compensatory strategies and
> a poor reader benefits more from direct methods
> that strengthen his weakness. Thus the dyslex-
> ic might be taught by the development of new
> skills to replace the deficient ones, while the

poor reader might be taught best by practice in the deficient skill itself.

Before examining the implications this might have for the teaching of Braille reading to blind children, it is worth turning to a third issue in intervention which is related to the direction that intervention might take. Practice in difficult or deficient skills often results in the experience of failure. There may be important motivational reasons for avoiding such failure. Cooper and Griffiths (1978) have made this point in regard to educational programmes for aphasic children. Noting that the language failure of such children is not due to a linguistically deprived environment, they point out that language enrichment and stimulation should not be the sole means of treatment. Children who are subjected to stimulation and demands beyond their abilities may react with disorganized, disturbed, or withdrawn behaviour.

What relevance do these last two issues have to the teaching of Braille reading to blind children? Millar has suggested that beginning Braille readers use a texture code and not a spatial one. Some of her results indicate that even older and better Braille readers continue to use a texture code to a great extent. Millar stresses the importance of spatial code training for Braille reading. Evidence has already been cited that blind individuals do not suffer from a spatial impairment, and thus the first issue raised in regard to intervention programmes for handicapped groups is not very important in the present context. However, the other two issues would seem to require some thought. It must first be adequately demonstrated that spatial coding is necessary for good Braille reading. Second, the finding by Millar that even good Braille readers appear to prefer texture coding needs to be explored. Since with other handicapped groups, intervention forcing a child to use a deficient or non-preferred system has motivational consequences that sometimes outweigh the advantages of such a programme, such issues must be adequately explored with the blind.

Millar's interesting case study and excellent experimental findings have given us pause to ponder a number of interesting issues concerning not only intervention programmes with the blind but with other handicapped groups as well. It is a measure of the worth of her ideas that they extend beyond the particulars of her studies with the blind.

Affolder, F., Bischofberger, W., Franklin, W. and
   Stockmann, I. (1980) Perceptual prerequisites for
   language development. *The Proceedings of the
   18th Congress of the International Association of
   Logopedics and Phoniatrics*. Washington D.C.
   pp. 163-7
Alich, G. (1960) *Zur Erkennbarkeit von Sprachgestal-
   ten beim Ablesen vom Munde*. Doctoral diss. of
   the University of Bonn, West Germany
Apkarian-Stielau, F. and Loomis, T.H. (1975) A com-
   parism of tactile and blurred visual form percep-
   tion. *Perception and Psychophysics, 18:* 362-8
Argyle, M. (1980) Die Sprache der Augen. *Der Sprach-
   heilpädagoge, 3:* 66-76
Atkinson, M. (1979) Prerequisites for reference. In
   E. Ochs and B.B. Schieffelin (eds.) *Developmental
   Pragmatics*. New York: Academic Press
Baddeley, A.D. (1976) *The psychology of memory*.
   New York: Harper and Row
Bartlett, E.J. (1978) The acquisition of the meaning
   of colour terms: a study of lexical development.
   In R.N. Campbell and P.T. Smith (eds.) *Recent
   advances in the psychology of language: language
   development and mother-child interaction*. New
   York: Plenum Press. pp. 89-108
Bates, E. (1976) *Language and context: the acquisi-
   tion of pragmatics*. New York: Academic Press
Bates, E., Benigni, L., Bretherton, I., Camaioni, L.
   and Volterra, V. (1977) *Cognition and communica-
   tion from 9-13 months: a correlational study*.
   Program on Cognitive and Perceptual Factors in
   Human Development Report #12. Institute for the
   study of Intellectual Behaviour, University of
   Colorado, Boulder

Bates, E., Camaioni, L. and Volterra, V. (1975) The
acquisition of performatives prior to speech.
Merrill Palmer Quarterly, 21: 205-26. Reprinted
in E. Ochs and B.B. Schieffelin (eds.) (1979)
Developmental pragmatics. New York: Academic
Press

Bateson, M.C. (1975) Mother-infant exchanges: the
epigenesis of conversational interaction. *Annals
of the New York Academy of Sciences, 263:* 101-13

Baumgarten, S. (1979) Zu den Begriffen Sprachstö-
rung, Sprachbehinderung, Sprachschädigung und
Sprachauffälligkeit. *Die Sprachheilarbeit, 24:*
67-77

Bayley, N. (1969) *Bayley scales of infant development.* New York: The Psychological Corporation

Beauvois, M.-F. (1981) Optic aphasia: a process of
interference between vision and language. Paper
presented at the conference, The Neuropsychology
of Cognitive Function, The Royal Society, London,
18-19 November 1981

Benesch, F. (1974) Ergebnisse der Erforschung kind-
licher Hirnschäden - Konsequenzen für den Bereich
der Blindenschule. *Der Blindenfreund, 6:* 141-8

Bernstein, D.K. (1980) *Semantic development in congenitally blind children.* Unpublished doctoral
diss., City University of New York

Blank, M. (1981) Verbal communication in hearing and
deaf pre-school children. Paper given at the
British Psychological Society Conference, Developmental Psychology Section, Manchester, Sept.
1981

Bloom, L. (1973) *One word at a time: the use of
single word utterances before syntax.* The Hague:
Mouton

Bloom, L., Lightbown, P. and Hood, L. (1975) Structure and variation in child language. *Monographs
of the Society for Research in Child Development,
40* (2)

Bowerman, M. (1973) *Early syntactic development: a
cross-linguistic study with special reference to
Finnish.* Cambridge: Cambridge University Press

Bowerman, M. (1978) The acquisition of word meaning:
an investigation into some current conflicts. In
N. Waterson and C. Snow (eds.) *The development of
communication.* Chichester: Wiley. pp. 263-87

Bracken, H.V. (1969) Mehrfachbehinderung als heilpädagogische Aufgabe. In H. Stutte and H.V.
Bracken (eds.) *Vernachlässigte Kinder. Heilpädagogische Forschung, 3. Beiheft.* Marburg:
Elwert

198

Brazelton, T.B., Koslowski, B. and Main, M. (1974)
The origins and reciprocity: the early mother-
infant interaction. In M. Lewis and L. Rosenblum
(eds.) *The effect of the infant on its caregiver.*
New York: Wiley. pp. 49-76

Brieland, D.M. (1950) A comparative study of the
speech of blind and sighted children. *Speech
Monographs, 17/1:* 99-103

Brown, R. (1973) *A first language: the early
stages.* Cambridge, Mass.: The University Press

Brown, R. (1977) Introduction. In C.E. Snow and
C. Ferguson (eds.) *Talking to children*
Cambridge: Cambridge University Press. pp. 1-27

Brown, R. and Hanlon, C. (1970) Derivational complexity and order of acquisition. In J. Hayes
(ed.) *Cognition and the development of language.*
New York: Wiley. pp. 11-53

Bruner, J.S. (1974/5) From communication to language - a psychological perspective. *Cognition,
3:* 255-87

Bruner, J.S. (1975) The ontogenesis of Speech Acts.
Journal of Child Language, 2: 1-19

Bruner, J.S. (1978) From communication to language:
a psychological perspective. In I. Markova (ed.)
The social context of language. Chichester:
Wiley. pp. 17-48

Burlingham, D. (1961) Some notes on the development
of the blind. *Psychoanalytic Study of the Child,
19:* 121-45

Burlingham, D. (1964) Hearing and its role in the
development of the blind. *Psychoanalytic Study
of the Child, 26:* 95-112

Carey, S. (1978) The child as word learner. In
M. Halle, J. Bresnan and G.A. Miller (eds.) *Lin-
guistic theory and psychological reality.*
Cambridge, Mass.: MIT Press. pp. 264-93

Carter, A. (1974) *The development of communication
in the sensorimotor period: a case study.* Unpublished doctoral diss., University of California, Berkeley

Carter, A. (1978) From sensori-motor vocalizations
to words: a case study of the evolution of attention-directing communication in the second
year. In A. Lock (ed.) *Action, gesture and
symbol: the emergence of language.* London:
Academic Press. pp. 309-51

Clahsen, H. (1981) *Der Erwerb der Syntax in der
frühen Kindheit.* Inaugural diss., Wuppertal, West
Germany

Clark, E.V. (1978) From gesture to word: on the natural history of deixis in language acquisition. In J.S. Bruner and A. Garton (eds.) *Human growth and development: Wolfson College Lectures 1976*. Oxford: The University Press. pp. 85-120

Clark, E.V. (1979) *The ontogenesis of meaning*. Wiesbaden: Adademische Verlagsgesellschaft Athenaion

Clark, E.V. and Clark, H. (1977) *Psychology and Language: an introduction to psycholinguistics*. New York: Harcourt Brace Jovanovich

Clark, R.A. (1978) The transition from action to gesture. In A. Lock (ed.) *Action, gesture and symbol: the emergence of language*. New York: Academic Press. pp. 231-60

Collis, G.M. and Schaffer, H.R. (1975) Synchronization of visual attention in mother-infant pairs. *Journal of Child Psychology, 16:* 315-20

Coltheart, M., Patterson, K. and Marshall, J.C. (eds.) (1980) *Deep dyslexia*. London: Routledge and Kegan Paul

Condon, W.S. and Sander, L.W. (1974) Synchrony demonstrated between movements of the neonate and adult speech. *Child Development, 45:* 456-62

Conrad, R. (1971) The chronology of the development of covert speech in children. *Developmental Psychology, 5:* 398-405

Conrad, R. (1979) *The deaf schoolchild*. New York: Harper and Row

Cooper, J.M. and Griffiths, P. (1978) Treatment and prognosis. In M.A. Wyke (ed.) *Developmental dysphasia*. London and New York: Academic Press. pp. 159-76

Cromer, R.F. (1973) Conservation by the congenitally blind. *British Journal of Psychology, 64:* 241-50

Cross, T. (1977) Mother's speech adjustments: the contribution of selected child listener variables. In C.E. Snow and C. Ferguson (eds.) *Talking to children: language input and acquisition*. Cambridge: Cambridge University Press. pp. 151-88

Crystal, D. (1980) *Introduction to language pathology*. London: Edward Arnold

Cutsforth, T.D. (1932) The unreality of words to the blind. *The Teachers Forum, 4:* 86-9

Cutsforth, T.D. (1951) *The blind in school and society*. New York: American Foundation for the Blind

Dodd, B. (1977) The role of vision in the perception of speech. *Perception, 6:* 31-40

Dodd, B. (1979) Lip reading in infants: attention to speech presented in- and out-of-synchrony. *Cognitive Psychology, 11:* 478-84

Dodd, B. (1980) Interaction of auditory and visual information in speech perception. *British Journal of Psychology, 71:* 541-9

Dodd, B. and Hermelin, B. (1977) Phonological coding by the prelinguistically deaf. *Perception and Psychophysics, 21:* 413-17

Dokecki, P.R. (1966) Verbalism and the blind, a critical view of the concepts and the literature. *Exceptional Children, 32:* 525-30

Donaldson, M. (1978) *Children's minds.* London: Fontana

Dore, J. (1974) A pragmatic description of early language development. *Journal of Psycholinguistic Research, 4:* 423-30

Dore, J. (1975) Holophrases, speech acts and language universals. *Journal of Child Language, 2:* 21-40

Dore, J. (1978) Conditions for the acquisition of speech acts. In I. Markova (ed.) *The social context of language.* Chichester: Wiley. pp. 87-112

Dore, J. (1979) Conversation and preschool language development. In P. Fletcher and M. Garman (eds.) *Language acquisition.* Cambridge: Cambridge University Press. pp. 337-61

Dressler, W.U. and Schaner-Wolles, C. (1981) Patholinguistik als Beitrag der Sprachwissenschaft zur Sprachheilarbeit. *Der Sprachheilpädagoge, 2:* 32-7

Edwards, D. (1973) Sensory-motor intelligence and semantic relations in early child grammar. *Cognition, 2:* 395-434

Elliot, A. (1981) *Child language.* Cambridge: Cambridge University Press

Elstner, W.(1955) Erfahrungen in der Behandlung sprachgestörter blinder Kinder. *Bericht über die Blindenlehrerfortbildungstagung in Innsbruck 1955.* Wien: Verlag des Bundes-Blindenerziehungsinstitutes. pp. 26-34

Elstner, W. (1966) Sprachstörungen bei blinden Kindern. *Der Blindenfreund, 86:* 33-41

Elstner, W. (1971) Blindheit und Sprachstörungen. *Heilpädagogische Forschung, 2:* 225-52.

Elstner, W. (1972) Rhythmische Erziehung sprachgeschädigter Kinder. In W. Orthmann (ed.) *Schulische Betreuung sprachbehinderter Kinder.* Berlin: Marhold. pp. 59-94

Erber, N.P. (1974) Visual perception of speech by deaf children: recent developments and

continuing needs. *Journal of Speech and Hearing Disorders, 39:* 178-85

Ewertsen, H.W. and Nielsen, H.B. (1971) A comparative analysis of the audiovisual, auditive and visual perception of speech. *Acta Otolarying, 72:* 201-5

Ferrier, L. (1978) Some observations of error in context. In N. Waterson and C.E. Snow (eds.) *The development of communication.* Chichester: Wiley. pp. 471-84

Fertsch, P. (1947) Hand dominance in reading Braille. *American Journal of Psychology, 60:* 335-49

Fisher, C.G. (1968) Confusions among visually perceived consonants. *Journal of Speech and Hearing Research, 11:* 796-804

Fiske, D. (1978) *Strategies for personality research, the observation versus interpretation of behavior.* San Francisco: Jossey-Bass

Fladeland Waterhouse, S.V. (1930) Some psychological effects of blindness as indicated by speech disorders. *Journal of Expression, 4*

Fodor, J.A. (1981) The present status of the innateness controversy. In J.A. Fodor (ed.) *Representations.* Cambridge, Mass.: MIT Press

Foulke, E. (1982) Reading Braille. In U. Schiff and E. Foulke (eds.) *Tactual perception: a sourcebook.* Cambridge: Cambridge University Press

Fraiberg, S. (1968) Parallel and divergent patterns in blind and sighted infants. *Psychoanalytic Study of the Child, 23:* 264-300

Fraiberg, S. (1974) Blind infants and their mothers: an examination of the sign system. In M. Lewis and A. Rosenblum (eds.) *The effects of the infant on its caregiver.* New York: Wiley and Sons. pp. 215-32

Fraiberg, S. (1977) *Insights from the blind: comparative studies of blind and sighted infants.* New York: Basic Books, and London: Souvenir Press

Fraiberg, S. and Adelson, E. (1975) Self-representation in language and play: observations of blind children. In E. Lenneberg and E. Lenneberg (eds.) *The foundations of language development: multi-disciplinary approach,* Vol. 2. New York: Academic Press. pp. 177-92

Frith, U. (1980) *Cognitive processes in spelling.* London: Academic Press

Frith, U. (1981) Experimental approaches to developmental dyslexia: an introduction. *Psychological Research, 43:* 97-109

Führing, M., Lettmayer, O., Elstner, W. and Lang, H.
(1981) *Die Sprachfehler des Kindes und ihre Be-
seitigung*. Wien: Österreichischer Bundesverlag.
8th edition

Furth, H. (1966) *Thinking without language*. New
York: Free Press

George, F. (1970) *Models of thinking*. (Advances in
Psychology: 1) London: George Allen and Unwin

Göllesz, V. (1972) Über die Lippenartikulation der
von Geburt an Blinden. *Papers in Interdisciplinary Speech Research*. Proceedings of the Speech
Symposium, Szeged,1971. Budapest: Akadéiai
Kiadó. pp. 85-91

Graham, M.D. (1968) *Multiply impaired blind children: a national problem*. New York: American
Foundation for the Blind

Greenfield, P. and Smith, J. (1976) *The structure of
communication in early language development*. New
York: Academic Press

Grice, H.P. (1975) The logic of conversation. In
P. Cole and J.L. Morgan (eds.) *Syntax and semantics 3: speech acts*. New York: Academic Press.
pp. 41-58

Halliday, M.A.K. (1973) *Explorations in the functions of language*. London: Arnold

Halliday, M.A.K. (1975a) Learning how to mean. In
E.H. Lenneberg and E. Lenneberg (eds.) *Foundations of language development: a multidiscipli-
nary approach*, Vol. 1. New York: Academic Press

Halliday, M.A.K. (1975b) *Learning how to mean*.
London: Arnold

Halliday, M.A.K. (1979) One child's protolanguage.
In M. Bullowa (ed.) *Before speech: the begin-
nings of interpersonal communication*. Cambridge:
Cambridge University Press

Harley, R. (1963) *Verbalism among blind children*.
New York: American Foundation for the Blind

Hartlage, L.C. (1976) Development of spatial concepts in visually deprived children. *Perceptual
and Motor Skills, 42*: 255-8

Häusler, R. (1968) *Sprachbehinderungen an Sonder-
schulen für Sehbehinderte und Blinde*. Unpublished dissertation at the Institut für Hör,-
Sprach- und Sehgeschädigtenlehrer in the Pädagogische Hochschule and University of Heidelberg

Hermelin, B. and O'Connor, N. (1971a) Functional
asymmetry in the reading of Braille. *Neuropsychologia, 9*: 431-5

Hermelin, B. and O'Connor, N. (1971b) Right and left
handed reading of Braille. *Nature, 231*: 470

Hermelin, B. and O'Connor, N. (1973) Ordering in recognition memory after ambiguous initial or recognition displays. *Canadian Journal of Psychology, 27:* 191-9

Herron, C.A. (1974) *A study of relational prepositions and their comprehension by blind and sighted children.* Honours thesis, Princeton University, USA.

Hess, M. (1959) *Die Sprachprüfung in der logopädischen Praxis.* Freiburg, Schweiz: Universitätsverlag

Hockett, C.F. (1960) The origin of speech. *Scientific American, 203:* 89-96

Homburg, G. (1981) Methodische Überlegungen zur therapeutischen Arbeit mit dysgrammatisch sprechenden Kindern. *Die Sprachheilarbeit, 26:* 267-81

Ihssen, W.B. (1977) Die Bedeutung von Linguistik, Psycholinguistik und Soziolinguistik für die Sprachbehindertenpädagogik. *Die Sprachheilarbeit, 22:* 165-76

Ihssen, W.B. (1978) Linguistik, Kindersprachforschung und Pathologie der Kindersprache. *Linguistische Berichte, 55:* 62-70

Ingram, D. (1976) *Phonological disability in children.* London: Edward Arnold

Jakobson, R. (1941) *Kindersprache, Aphasie und allgemeine Lautgesetze.* Frankfurt a.M.: Suhrkamp, 1969. Translated as *Child language, aphasia and phonological universals.* The Hague: Mouton, 1968

Jorm, A.F. (1979) The cognitive and neurological basis of developmental dyslexia: a theoretical framework and review. *Cognition, 7:* 19-33

Karmiloff-Smith, A. (1979) Language development after five. In P.J. Fletcher and M. Garman (eds.) *Language acquisition.* Cambridge: Cambridge University Press. pp. 307-23

Kaye, K. (1977) Towards the origin of dialogue. In H.R. Schaffer (ed.) *Studies of mother-infant interaction.* London: Academic Press

Keenan, E.O. and Schieffelin, B.B. (1976) Topic as a discourse notion: a study of topic in the conversations of children and adults. In Ch.N. Li (ed.) *Subject and topic.* New York: Academic Press. pp. 335-84

Kephart, J.G., Kephart, C.P. and Schwarz, G.G. (1974) A journey into the world of the blind child. *Exceptional Children, 40:* 421-7

Kiphart, E. (1972) Sensomotorische Entwicklungshilfen. *Der Blindenfreund, 92:* 52-60

Kostjutschek, N.S. (1974) *Die Entwicklung der Sprache bei blinden Kindern*. Institut für Defektologie der Akademie der Pädagogischen Wissenschaften, Moscow

Kruse, E. (1980) Zentrale Sprachentwicklungsstörungen - Differentialdiagnose und Therapie. *Die Sprachheilarbeit, 25/6*: 205-12

Kubiak, I. (1979) Spracherziehung bei 3- bis 5-jährigen Kinder mit HSR. *Die Sonderschule, 24/6*: 362-71

Labov, W. and Fanshel, D. (1977) *Therapeutic discourse*. New York: Academic Press

Landau, B. (1982) *Language learning in blind children: relationships between perception and language*. Unpublished doctoral diss., University of Pennsylvania

Landau, B. and Gleitman, L.R. (in prep.) *Language development and the language of perception in blind babies*. Manuscript, University of Pennsylvania

Landau, B., Gleitman, H. and Spelke, E. (1981) Spatial inference and geometric representation in a child blind from birth. *Science, 213*: 1275-8

Leech, G. (1971) *Meaning and the English verb*. London: Longman

Leischner, A. (1967) Die Sprachstörungen im Kindesalter. *Zeitschrift für Kinderheilkunde, 100*: 137-59

Lenneberg, E.H. (1967) *Biological foundations of language*. New York: Wiley

Leopold, W. (1949) *Speech development of a bilingual child, Vol. 3, Grammar and general problems*. Evanston: Northwestern University Press

Lewis, M. and Rosenblum, L.A. (eds.) (1977) *Interaction, conversation and the development of language*. New York: Wiley

Liberman, A.M., Cooper, F.S., Shankweiler, D.P. and Studdert Kennedy, M. (1967) Perception of the speech code. *Psychological Review, 74*: 431-61

Linck, H.A. and Haberkamp, H. (1976) Sprachentwicklungsbehinderung - Sprachentwicklungsverzögerung, Versuch einer Abgrenzung. *Folia Phoniatrica, 28*: 141-60

Locke, J. (1690) An essay concerning human understanding. Reprinted in *The Empiricists*. New York: Anchor Press, 1974

Lopata, D.J. and Pasnak, R. (1976) Accelerated conservation acquisition and IQ gains by blind children. *Genetic Psychology Monographs, 93*: 3-25

Lux, G. (1933) Eine Untersuchung über die nachteilige Wirkung des Ausfalls der optischen

Perzeption auf die Sprache des Blinden. *Der Blindenfreund, 53:* 166-70

Lyons, J. (1975) Deixis as a source of reference. In E.L. Keenan (ed.) *Formal semantics of natural language.* Cambridge: Cambridge University Press. pp. 61-83

MacDonald, J. and McGurk, H. (1978) Visual influences on speech perception processes. *Perception and Psychophysics, 24:* 253-7

McGurk, H. and Buchanan, L. (1981) *Bimodal speech perception: vision and hearing.* Unpublished paper, University of Surrey

McGurk, H. and MacDonald, J. (1976) Hearing lips and seeing voices. *Nature, 264:* 746-8

McGurk, H. and MacDonald, J. (1977) *Hearing lips and seeing voices: a new illusion.* Paper to the Annual Conference of the British Psychological Society, University of Exeter

McShane, J. (1980) *Learning to talk.* Cambridge: Cambridge University Press

McTear, M. (1978) Review of Snow and Ferguson (eds.) Talking to children. *Journal of Child Language, 5:* 521-30

Mansfeld, F. (1952) Die Lehre Arnold Gehlens von den Kreisprozessen und ihre Bedeutung für das Blindenwesen. *Der Blindenfreund, 72/2:* 35-51

Marshall, J.C. and Newcombe, F. (1973) Patterns of paralexia: a psycholinguistic approach. *Journal of Psycholinguistic Research, 2:* 175-99

Marshall, J.C. and Newcombe, F. (1977) Variability and constraint in acquired dyslexia. In H. Whitaker and H.A. Whitaker (eds.) *Studies in neurolinguistics, Vol. 3.* New York: Academic Press. pp. 257-86

Maxfield, K.E. (1928) *The blind child and his reading.* New York: American Foundation for the Blind

Menyuk, P. (1964) Comparison of grammar of children with functionally deviant and normal speech. *Journal of Speech and Hearing Research, 7:* 107-21

Menyuk, P. (1969) *Sentences children use.* Cambridge, Mass.: MIT Press

Millar, S. (1975) Effects of tactual and phonological similarity on the recall of Braille letters by blind children. *British Journal of Psychology, 66:* 193-201

Millar, S. (1977a) Early stages of tactual matching. *Perception, 6:* 333-43

Millar, S. (1977b) Tactual and name matching by blind children. *British Journal of Psychology, 68:* 377-83

Millar, S. (1978a) Short-term serial tactual recall:
effects on grouping tactually probed recall of
Braille letters and nonsense shapes by blind
children. *British Journal of Psychology, 69:*
17-24

Millar, S. (1978b) Aspects of memory for information
from touch and movement. In G. Gordon (ed.)
Active touch. Oxford: Pergamon Press. pp. 215-
27

Millar, S. (1981) Crossmodal and intersensory perception and the blind. In R.D. Walk and
H.L. Pick Jr. (eds.) *Intersensory perception and
sensory integration.* London: Plenum Press

Miller, G. (1967) Information and memory. In
G. Miller (ed.) *The psychology of communication.*
Harmondsworth: Penguin Press. pp. 3-13

Miller, G. and Johnson-Laird, P. (1976) *Language and
perception.* Cambridge: Cambridge University
Press

Miller, G. and Nicely, P.E. (1955) An analysis of
perceptual confusions among some English consonants. *Journal of the Acoustical Society of
America, 27:* 338-52

Miller, M. (1976) Zur Logik der frühkindlichen
Sprachentwicklung. Stuttgart: Klett

Miller, M. and Weissenborn, J. (1979) Pragmatische
Voraussetzungen für den Erwerb lokaler Referenz.
In K. Martens (ed.) *Kindliche Kommunikation.*
Frankfurt: Suhrkamp. pp. 61-75

Mills, A.E. (1978) *Visual information and imitation
in child language.* Paper to the Child Language
Seminar, York, England

Mills, A.E. (to appear) The acquisition of German.
In D.I. Slobin (ed.) *The crosslinguistic study of
language acquisition.* Hillsdale, New Jersey:
Erlbaum

Mills, A.E. and Thiem, R. (1980) Auditory-visual
fusions and illusions in speech perception.
Linguistische Berichte, 68/80: 85-108

Milner, B. (1971) Interhemispheric differences in
the localization of psychological processes in
man. *British Medical Bulletin, 27:* 272

Miner, L.E. (1963) A study of the incidence of
speech deviations among visually handicapped
children. *New Outlook for the Blind, 57:* 10-14

Mulford, R.C. (1981) *Talking without seeing: some
problems of semantic development in blind children.* Unpublished doctoral diss., Stanford
University

Murphy, C. and Messer, D. (1977) Mother, infants,
and the pointing gesture. In H.R. Schaffer (ed.)

Studies in mother-infant interaction. London:
Academic Press
Neilson, I. (1981) *Visual development in the 'blind'
child.* Paper given at the British Psychological
Society Conference, Developmental Psychology
Section, Manchester, Sept. 1981
Nelson, K. (1973) Structure and strategy in learning
to talk. *Monographs of the Society for Research
in Child Development, 38* (Serial No. 149)
Nelson, K. (1978) Semantic development and the de-
velopment of semantic memory. In K.E. Nelson
(ed.) *Children's language, Vol. 1.* New York:
Gardner Press. pp. 39-80
Nolan, C.Y. (1960) On the unreality of words to the
blind. *New Outlook for the Blind, 54:* 100-2
Nolan, C.Y. and Kederis, C.J. (1969) *Perceptual fac-
tors in Braille word recognition.* New York:
American Foundation for the Blind
Norris, M., Spaulding, P.J. and Brodie, F.H. (1957)
Blindness in children. Chicago: University of
Chicago Press
Ochs, E., Schieffelin, B.B. and Platt, M.L. (1979)
Propositions across utterances and speakers. In
E. Ochs and B.B. Schieffelin (eds.) *Developmental
pragmatics.* New York: Academic Press. pp. 251-
68
O'Connor, N. and Hermelin, B. (1973a) Short-term
memory for the order of pictures and syllables by
deaf and hearing children. *Neuropsychologia, 11:*
437-42
O'Connor, N. and Hermelin, B. (1973b) The spatial or
temporal organization of short-term memory.
Quarterly Journal of Experimental Psychology, 25:
335-43
O'Connor, N. and Hermelin, B. (1978) *Seeing and
hearing and space and time.* London: Academic
Press
Oléron, P. (1950) *Recherches sur le développement
mental de sourds muets.* Paris
Oller, D.K. and Kelly, C.A. (1974) Phonological substitution processes of a hard-of-hearing child.
Journal of Speech and Hearing Disorders, 39:
65-74
O'Neill, J.J. (1954) Contributions of the visual
components of oral symbols to speech comprehen-
sion. *Journal of Speech and Hearing Disorders,
19:* 429-39
Ortony, A. (ed.) (1979) *Metaphor and thought.*
Cambridge: Cambridge University Press
Pavlovitch, M. (1920) *Le langage enfantin:
acquisition du serbe et du français par un enfant*

serbe. Paris: Champion

Pechmann, T. and Deutsch, W. (1980) From gesture to word and gesture. *Papers and Reports on Child Language Development, 19:* 113-20

Peuser, G. (1978) *Aphasie. Eine Einführung in die Patholinguistik*. Munich: Fink

Piaget, J. (1951) *Play, dreams and imitation*. London: Routledge and Kegan-Paul

Piaget, J. (1953) *The origins of intelligence in the child*. London: Routledge and Kegan-Paul

Piaget, J. (1955) *The child's construction of reality*. London: Routledge and Kegan-Paul

Piaget, J. and Inhelder, B. (1969) *The psychology of the child*. London: Routledge and Kegan-Paul

Provence, S. and Lipton, R. (1962) *Infants in institutions*. New York: International Universities Press

Rieder, K. (1980) Angewandte Sprachwissenschaft und Sprachheilpädagogik. *Der Sprachheilpädagoge, 4:* 2-10

Rogow, S.M. (1972) Language acquisition and the blind retarded child: a study of impaired communication. *Education of the Visually Handicapped:* 36-40

Rogow, S.M. (1973) Speech development and the blind multi-impaired child. *Education of the Visually Handicapped:* 105-9

Ronjat, J. (1913) *Le développement du langage observé chez un enfant bilingue*. Paris: Champion

Rosch, E. (1977) Linguistic relativity. In P.N. Johnson-Laird and P.C. Wason (eds.) *Thinking: readings in cognitive science*. Cambridge: Cambridge University Press. pp. 501-19

Ross, J.R. (1972) Act. In D. Davidson and G. Harman (eds.) *The semantics of natural language*. Dordrecht: D. Reidel. pp. 70-126

Rowland, C.M. (1980) *Communicative strategies of visually impaired infants and their mothers*. Unpublished doctoral diss., University of Oklahoma

Rowland, C.M. (1981) Communicative strategies of visually impaired infants and their mothers: descriptive data. In B. Urban (ed.) *Proceedings of the 18th Congress of the International Association of Logopedics and Phoniatrics*. American Speech- Language and Hearing Association. pp. 87-92

Rutter, M., Tizard, J. and Whitmore, K. (eds.) (1970) *Education, health and behaviour*. London: Longman

Rutter, M., Tizard, J., Yule, W., Graham, P. and Whitmore, K. (1976) Research report: Isle of

Wight studies 1964-1974. *Psychological Medicine, 6:* 313-32

Rutter, M. and Yule, W. (1975) The concept of specific reading retardation. *Journal of Child Psychology and Psychiatry, 16:* 181-97

Sachs, H., Schegloff, E. and Jefferson, G. (1974) A simplest systematics for the organisation of turntaking for conversation. *Language, 50:* 696-735

Sachs, J. (1977) Talking about there and then. *Papers and Reports on Child Language Development, 13:* 56-63

Sackett, G.P. (1979) The lag sequential analysis of contingency and cyclicity in behavioral interaction research. In J.D. Osofsky (ed.) *Handbook of infant development.* New York: Wiley

Sackett, G.P. (1980) Lag sequential analysis as a data reduction technique in social interaction research. In D.B. Sawin, R.C. Hawkins, L.O. Walker and J.H. Penticuff (eds.) *Exceptional Infant, Vol. 4: psychosocial risks in infant-environment transactions.* New York: Brunner-Mazel. pp. 300-40

Schaffer, H.R. (ed.) (1977) *Studies in mother-infant interaction.* London: Academic Press

Schiefelbusch, R.L. and Lloyd, L.L. (eds.) (1978) *Language perspectives, retardation and intervention.* Baltimore: University Park Press

Scholz, H.-J. (1970) Von der Notwendigkeit linguo-diagnostischer Verfahren für die Zeit der Sprachentwicklung. *Die Sprachheilarbeit, 15/4:* 97-103

Scupin, E. and Scupin, G. (1907) *Bubis erste Kindheit, Vol 1.* Leipzig: Th. Griebens Verlag

Semzowa, M.I. (1961) Besonderheiten der Erkenntnistätigkeit blinder Kinder im jüngeren Schulalter. *Die Sonderschule, 6/6:* 336-40 and *7/1:* 29-38

Semzowa, M.I. and Solnzewa, L.I. (1966) Die psychologisch-pädagogische Untersuchung blinder Schulanfänger. *Die Sonderschule, 11/5:* 279-83 and *11/6:* 344-51

Sinclair-de Zwart (1969) Developmental psycholinguistics. In D. Elkind and J.H. Flavell (eds.) *Studies in cognitive development.* Oxford: Oxford University Press. pp. 315-36

Sinclair-de Zwart (1970) The transition from sensory motor behaviour to symbolic activity. *Interchange, 1:* 119-26

Slobin, D.I. (1973) Cognitive prerequisites for the development of grammar. In C. Ferguson and D.I. Slobin (eds.) *Studies in child language development.* New York: Holt, Rinehart and Winston. pp. 175-276

Slobin, D.I. (1978) *Universal and particular in the acquisition of language*. Paper presented at the workshop-conference "Language acquisition: state of the art", University of Pennsylvania, May 19-22, 1978

Smith, M., Chethik, M. and Adelson, E. (1969) Differential assessment of "blindisms". *American Journal of Orthopsychiatry, 39/5:* 807-17

Smith, N.V. (1973) *The acquisition of phonology.* Cambridge: Cambridge University Press

Snow, C. (1977a) Mother's speech research: from input to interaction. In C. Snow and C. Ferguson (eds.) *Talking to children: language, input and acquisition.* Cambridge: Cambridge University Press. pp. 1-27

Snow, C. (1977b) The development of conversation between mothers and babies. *Journal of Child Language, 4/1:* 1-22

Snowling, M.J. (1980) The development of grapheme-phoneme correspondence in normal and dyslexic readers. *Journal of Experimental Child Psychology, 29:* 294-305

Solnzewa, L.I. (1975) Die Besonderheiten in der Entwicklung des blinden Vorschulkindes. *Die Sonderschule, 20/5:* 304-8

Solnzewa, L.I. (1977) Die Besonderheiten der psychischen Entwicklung blinder Kinder. *Die Sonderschule, 22/2:* 104-10

Solnzewa, L.I. (1980) Kompensation der Blindheit im Kleinkindalter. *Die Sonderschule, 25/1:* 34-9

Solnzewa, L.I. (1981) Kompensation der Blindheit in der frühen Kindheit. *Die Sonderschule, 26/4:* 228-34

Sperber, D. (1975) *Rethinking symbolism.* Cambridge: Cambridge University Press. (Originally published in French in 1974.)

Stern, D.N. (1974) Mother and infant at play: the dyadic interaction involving facial, vocal and gaze behaviors. In M. Lewis and L. Rosenblum (eds.) *The effect of the infant on its caregiver.* New York: Wiley. pp. 187-214

Stern, D.N., Jaffe, J., Beebe, R. and Bennett, S.L. (1975) Vocalizing in unison and in alternation: two modes of communication within the mother-infant dyad. *Annals of the New York Academy of Sciences, 263:* 89-99

Stillman, R.S. (ed.) (1978) *The Callier-Azusa Scale.* Dallas, Texas: Callier Center for Communication Disorders

Stinchfield, S.M. (1928) *Speech pathology.* Mogrilia, Mass.: Expression Company

Sumby, W.H. and Pollack, J. (1954) Visual contribution to speech intelligibility in noise. *Journal of the Acoustical Society of America, 26:* 212-15

Summerfield, Q. (1979) Use of visual information for phonetic perception. *Phonetica, 36:* 314-31

Tervoort, B. (1972) The understanding of passive sentences by normal, deaf and hard-of-hearing children. In *Proceedings of the VIth Congress of Applied Linguistics.* Heidelberg

Tervoort, B. (1981) *Mother-deaf child interaction.* Unpublished paper, University of Amsterdam

Thimm, W. (1977) Soziale Rahmenbedingungen der Sondererziehung und Rehabilitation Sehgeschädigter. *Der Blindenfreund, 97/3/4:* 74-83

Trevarthen, C. (1974) Conversation with a two-month-old. *New Scientist, 62:* 230

Trevarthen, C. and Hubley, P. (1978) Secondary intersubjectivity: confidence, confiding and acts of meaning in the first year. In A. Lock (ed.) *Action, gesture and symbol: the emergence of language.* London: Academic Press. pp. 183-231

Tronick, E.D., Als, H. and Brazelton, T.B. (1977) Mutuality in mother-infant interactions. *Journal of Communication, 27:* 74-9

Urwin, C. (1978a) *The development of communication between blind infants and their parents: some ways into language.* Unpublished doctoral diss., University of Cambridge, England.

Urwin, C. (1978b) Early language development in blind children. *British Psychological Society Occasional Papers, 2/2:* 73-87

Urwin, C. (1978c) The development of communication between blind infants and their parents. In A. Lock (ed.) *Action, gesture, symbol: the emergence of language.* London: Academic Press. pp. 79-108

Urwin, C. (1979) Preverbal communication and early language development in blind children. In *Papers and Reports on Child Language Development, 17:* 119-28

van der Geest, T. (1977) Some interactional aspects of language acquisition. In C. Snow and C. Ferguson (eds.) *Talking to children.* Cambridge: Cambridge University Press. pp. 89-107

van der Geest, T. (1978) Mother-child interaction and their researchers. *Grazer linguistische Studien, 10:* 46-69

van der Geest, T. (1981) Psychologische aspecten van taalwetenschappelijk onderzoek. In M. Steehouder (ed.) *Taalbeheersingsonderzoek.* VIOT. pp. 200-12

van der Geest, T. and Heckhausen, J. (1981) Kommuni-
kative Anpassung zwischen Kindern verschiedenen
Alters und verschiedener Muttersprache. *Zeitschrift für Entwicklungspsychologie und Pädagogische Psychologie, 13:* 83-105

Vygotsky, L.S. (1962) *Thought and language.*
Cambridge, Mass.: MIT Press, and New York:
Wiley. (Originally published in Russian in 1934)

Walden, B.E., Prosek, R.A., Montgomery, A.A.,
Scherr, C.K. and Jones, C.J. (1977) Effects of
training on the visual recognition of consonants.
Journal of Speech and Hearing Research, 20: 130-
45

Walkerdine, V. and Corran, G. (1979) *Cognitive development: a mathematical experience?* Paper
presented at the British Psychological Society
Conference, Developmental Section on Social
Cognition, Southampton, Sept. 1979

Walkerdine, V. and Sinha, C. (1978) The internal
triangle: language, reasoning and the social
context. In I. Markova (ed.) *The social context
of language.* Chichester: Wiley. pp. 151-76

Warren, D.H. (1977) *Blindness and early childhood
development.* New York: American Foundation for
the Blind.

Wason, P.C. and Johnson-Laird, P.N. (1972) *Psychology of reasoning: structure and content.* London:
Batsford

Werth, P. (1981) The concept of 'rele nce' in conversational analysis. In P. Werth (' *Conversation and discourse: structure and i.   reta-
tion.* London: Croom Helm. pp. 129-54

Wexler, K. and Culicover, P. (1980) *Formal pri.
ples of language acquisition.* Cambridge, Mas.
MIT Press

White, R.W. (1959) Motivation re-considered: the
concept of competence. *Psychological Review,
66:* 297-333

Williams, M. (1956) *Williams intelligence test for
children with defective vision.* Reading:
N.F.E.R. Publishing Company

Wills, D.M. (1970) Vulnerable periods in the early
development of blind children. *Psychoanalytic
Study of the Child, 25:* 461-80

Wills, D.M. (1978) Early speech development in blind
children. *The Psychoanalytic Study of the Child,
34:* 85-117

Wilson, D. and Sperber, D. (1981) On Grice's theory
of conversation. In P. Werth (ed.) *Conversation
and discourse: structure and interpretation.*
London: Croom Helm. pp. 155-178

Wode, H. (1977) Four early stages in the development of L1 negation. *Journal of Child Language, 4:* 87-102

Wode, H. (1981) *Learning a second language. I. An integrated view of language acquisition.* Tübingen: Narr

Wood, M. (1970) *Problems in the development and home care of preschool blind children.* Unpublished doctoral diss., University of Nottingham, England

Woodward, M.F. and Barber, C.G. (1960) Phoneme perception in lipreading. *Journal of Speech and Hearing Research, 3:* 212-22

Wundt, W. (1911) *Völkerpsychologie Bd. I: Die Sprache.* Leipzig: Engelman. 3rd ed.

Young, E.H. and Hawk, S.S. (1955) *Moto-kinesthetic speech training.* Stanford, California: Stanford University Press

AUTHOR INDEX

Adelson, E.	1-12, 13, 16, 111, 128, 144-6
Affolder, F.	39
Alich, G.	46
Als, H.	124
Apkarian-Stielau, F.	172
Argyle, M.	19
Atkinson, M.	89, 91, 95
Baddeley, A.D.	184
Barber, C.G.	46
Bartlett, E.J.	189
Bates, E.	89, 94, 106, 115-6, 128, 130-1, 143-4, 149
Bateson, M.C.	127
Baumgarten, S.	24
Bayley, N.	64
Beauvois, M.-F.	189
Beebe, R.	124
Benesch, F.	27, 36
Bennett, S.L.	124
Bernstein, D.K.	104
Blank, M.	112
Bleuler, R.	36
Bloom, L.	66, 76, 143
Bowerman, M.	89, 96, 142-3, 149
Bracken, H.V.	26
Brazelton, T.B.	124, 144
Brieland, D.M.	26
Brodie, F.H.	64, 90
Brown, R.	134, 136, 142-3, 151
Bruner, J.S.	62, 89, 95, 115, 128, 134, 143-4, 150, 162
Buchanan, L.	47
Burlingham, D.	114, 144

Camaioni, L.   94, 143
Carey, S.   188, 189
Carter, A.   95, 143-4
Chethik, M.   4
Clahsen, H.   133-4, 137
Clark, E.V.   77, 89, 96, 106, 156
Clark, H.   77
Clark, R.A.   115
Collis, G.M.   110, 144, 150
Coltheart, M.   170
Condon, W.S.   124
Conrad, R.   170, 173
Cooper, J.   196
Corran, G.   147, 161
Cromer, R.F.   144, 187-196
Cross, T.   153
Culicover, P.   63
Cutsforth, T.D.   63, 75, 104, 161
Crystal, D.   43

Deutsch, W.   96
Dodd, B.   47, 57-61, 110
Dokecki, P.R.   104
Donaldson, M.   146
Dore, J.   115, 143, 162
Dressler, W.U.   42

Edwards, D.   142, 143
Ellist, A.   146, 160
Elstner, W.   18-41, 42-44, 56, 59,
                                        108, 112, 114, 145,
                                        163
Erber, N.P.   46
Ewertsen, H.W.   47

Fanshel, D.   136
Ferrier, L.   149
Fertsch, P.   175
Fisher, C.G.   46
Fiske, D.   136, 140
Fladeland-Waterhouse, S.V.   23
Fodor, J.A.   74
Foulke, E.   172, 180, 184
Fraiberg, S.   1, 4, 12, 18-19, 22,
                                        26, 62, 90, 106,
                                        114, 128, 137, 144-6
                                        150, 156
Frith, U.   170, 195
Führing, M.   39
Furth, H.   137

Garman, M.   162-6
George, F.   81
Gleitman, H.   73
Gleitman, L.R.   63, 73, 75
Göllesz, V.   23
Graham, M.D.   36-7, 114
Greenfield, P.   151
Grice, H.P.   86
Griffiths, P.   196

Haberkamp, H.   37
Halliday, M.A.K.   89, 115, 143
Hanlon, C.   134
Harley, R.   104
Hartlage, L.C.   131
Hatwell, P.   137
Häusler, O.   23-5, 28, 40
Hawk, S.S.   36-7
Heckhausen, J.   134
Hermelin, B.   61, 191-3
Herron, C.A.   104
Hess, M.   28, 31
Hockett, C.F.   88
Homburg, G.   39
Hood, L.   66, 76
Hubley, P.   144
Huxley   152

Ihssen, W.B.   40, 43
Ingram, D.   15
Inhelder, B.   144

Jaffe, J.   124
Jakobson, R.   14
Jefferson, G.   149
Johnson-Laird, P.N.   77-8, 81, 86
Jorm, A.F.   194

Karmiloff-Smith, A.   96
Kaye, K.   110
Kederis, C.J.   172
Keenan, E.O.   91, 94
Kelly, C.A.   61
Kephart, C.P.   131
Kephart, J.G.   131
Kiphard, E.   39
Knolke   36
Koslowski, B.   144
Kostjutschek, N.S.   23
Kruse, E.   37
Kubiak, I.   40

Labov, W.	136
Landau, B.	15, 62-76, 79-81, 84-5, 104, 108, 112, 144, 159, 187
Lang, H.	39
Leischner, A.	37
Leech, G.	82
Lenneberg, E.H.	43
Leopold, W.	14
Lettmayer, O.	39
Lewis, M.	115
Liberman, A.M.	61
Lightbown, P.	66, 76
Linck, H.A.	37
Lipton, R.	4-5
Lloyd, L.L.	40
Locke, J.	74
Loomis, T.H.	131, 172
Lopata, D.J.	131
Lux, G.	20, 23, 40
Lyons, J.	89
MacDonald, J.	47, 57, 61, 159
McGurk, H.	47, 57, 61, 108-13, 149, 159, 164
McShane, J.	146
McTear, M.	136
Main, M.	144
Mansfeld, F.	21
Marshall, J.C.	193
Maxfield, K.E.	24
Menyuk, P.	43
Messer, D.	111
Millar, S.	104, 167-86, 187, 190, 192-3, 196
Miller, G.A.	40, 46-7, 77-8, 81, 86
Miller, M.	134
Mills, A.E.	15, 23, 40, 43, 46-56, 57, 59-60, 110, 142, 159
Milner, B.	174
Miner, L.E.	24-5, 114
Mulford, R.C.	15, 89-107, 130, 163
Murphy, C.	111
Neilson, I.	113
Nelson, K.	64, 76, 95, 142, 145, 188
Newcombe, F.	193
Nicely, P.E.	46-7
Nielson, H.B.	47

Nolan, C.Y.   104, 172
Norris, M.   5, 64, 89

Ochs, E.   89, 91, 94, 97
O'Connor, N.   61, 191-3
Oléran, P.   137
Oller, D.K.   61
O'Neill, J.J.   46
Ortony, A.   161

Pasnak, R.   131
Pavlovitch, M.   14
Pechmann, T.   96
Peuser, G.   45
Piaget, J.   14, 16-17, 89, 134-5,
                                   137, 142, 144-6.
Platt, M.L.   89
Pollack, J.   46
Provence, S.   4-5

Rieder, K.   44
Rogow, S.M.   19, 21, 23, 36-7
Ronjat, J.   14
Rosch, E.   189
Rosenblum, L.A.   115
Ross, J.R.   84
Rowland, C.M.   90, 100, 106-7, 114-32,
                                   133, 135, 137-8, 142,
                                   149
Rutter, M.   195

Sachs, H.   149
Sachs, J.   96
Sackett, G.P.   124
Sander, L.W.   124
Schaffer, H.R.   110, 115, 143-4, 150
Schaner-Wolles, C.   15, 42-5, 108
Schegloff, E.   149
Schiefelbusch, R.L.   40
Schieffelin, B.   89, 91, 94
Scholz, H.-J.   35, 39
Schwarz, G.G.   131
Scupin, E.   49
Scupin, G.   49
Semzowa, M.I.   20, 25
Sinclair-de Zwart, H.   134, 137
Sinha, C.   146
Slobin, D.I.   134, 143, 190
Smith, J.   151
Smith, M.   4, 151
Smith, N.V.   50

Snow, C. 153
Snowling, M.J. 194
Solnzewa, L.I. 18-21, 23, 25
Spaulding, P. 5, 64, 89
Spelke, E. 73
Sperber, D. 86, 188
Stern, D.N. 124, 144
Stillmann, R.S. 116
Stinchfield, S.M. 24-5
Sumby, W.H. 46
Summerfield, Q. 47

Tervoort, B. 137, 141
Thiem, R. 23, 47-8, 57
Thimm, W. 35
Trevarthen, C. 22, 144
Tronick, E.D. 124

Urwin, C. 15, 101, 106-7, 130, 137, 142-161, 162, 164-5

van der Geest, T. 133-141, 142
Volterra, V. 94, 143
Vygotsky, L.S. 189

Walden, B.E. 46, 51
Walkerdine, V. 146-7, 161
Warren, D.H. 63, 69
Wason, P.C. 81
Weissenborn, J. 134
Werth, P. 77-88, 144, 188
Wexler, K. 63
White, R.W. 110
Williams, M. 175, 179
Wills, D.M. 18-23, 26, 145-6, 150
Wilson, D. 86
Wode, H. 13-17, 109
Wood, M. 145
Woodward, M.F. 46
Wundt, W. 49

Yoder, D. 40
Young, E.H. 36-7
Yule, W. 195

abnormalities, see
   language abnormali-
   ties, phonological ab-
   normalities, speech
   abnormalities, verbal
   communication
abstract representation
   71
abstract thought 12
acoustic information 49,
   56
action words 64, 66, 82,
   84
acquisition, see first
   language acquisition,
   language acquisition,
   language development,
   nouns, personal-social
   words, questions, syntax
addressee 62, 90, 98
affection 19
affective ties 1
agrammatism 33
aniridia 147
anopthalmia 117
aphasia 45
aphasic children 196
aphasic patients
   reading 193
articulation 23, 40, 46,
   56
   disorders 43
   manner of 47-8, 59
   place of 47, 59
articulatory mistakes 22
articulatory movements
   46-7, 49, 55
articulatory positions
   48, see also articu-
   lation, lip move-
   ments, visually dis-
   tinctive sounds
assessment
   language 164-5
   see also diagnosis,
   speech therapy,
   verbal tests
assimulation 56, see
   also phonological
   rules
attachment, human 2, 4
   see also affection,
   affective ties,
   emotional ties
attention
   assessing in listener
      91-2, 94, 97-9,
      101-2, 105-6, 165
   attracting to self
      92, 94, 99-101,
      130
   confirmation of
      listener's 99
   directing to referent
      95-6, 102-3, 130,
      143
   distant object 150
   focus of 94, 110
   infants 110, 148-9
   mutual 144, 150, 153,
      155
   see also regard,

gaze, pointing, referential development, touching
audition 61
  code 61
  verbs 72
auditory cues 57
  eye orientation to 116
  head turn to 116
auditory information 23,
    47-8, 58, 127
  processing 46
auditory localization
    skills 116, see also
  reach on sound
auditory modality 49, 57
auditory perception 21, 39
auditory presentation 194
auditory stimulus 60
auditory threshold
  sighted children 20
  blind children 20
Austria 29, 44

babbling 9-11, 22, 116
behaviours
  caretaking 110
  communicative 115, 120,
    147
  compensatory 19
  dead-end 4
  infant 115, 119, 120,
    125, 135
  maternal 115, 120
  non-verbal 111
  pre-verbal 115, 127
blind adult 66, 106, 164
blind children
  cognitive development
    114, 131, 137-8,
    142, 144
  crawling 4-5, 7, 9-10
  development of communi-
    cative competence
    112-3
  expressed meanings 64-9
  gesture 121-9, 131, 146,
    153
  imitation 20-2, 118-19,
    121, 128-9, 145, 149
  interaction 106, 114-33,

136, 150-1, 153
  language development
    12, 34, 56, 59,
    131, 162
  lexical development
    149
  manual activity 116,
    121, 123
  parents 106, 111,
    147-51
  phonological devel-
    opment 22-3,
    55-6, 60
  reading 167-86
  referential develop-
    ment 89-107
  speech therapy 22,
    27, 39-40, 42-5,
    56
  walking 4, 7, 9,
    11-12
  see also congenital-
    ly blind, partially-
    sighted children,
    totally blind
blind children studied
  Alex 97, 99-100,
    102-3
  Amy 116-8, 122-6,
    130
  Angie 64, 76
  Carlo 64, 66
  Hanna 50-56
  Helen 175-186
  Jerry 147-8, 158
  Joshua 97-100, 103,
    105
  Karen 2-13
  Kelli 64, 66, 69-81,
    84, 86-7
  Maria 116-8, 122-131
    137
  Nicola 59
  Robert 97-101, 103
  Steven 148, 151, 158
  Suzanne 147-61, 165
  Tanya 116, 119,
    122-6, 128, 130
blindism 10
blindness
  awareness of 73

handicap 72, 88, 134
  nature of 75
  see also handicap,
  vision, visual im-
  pairment
Braille 40, 173-8, 184
  hand advantage in
    174-5, 193
Braille keyboard
  Perkins 176, 181
Braille reading 170-87,
  190-6
  models of 171-2, 181-5
  retardation in 170,
    175, 178-80
  spatial coding 170,
    175-6, 178-81, 186,
    190-3, 196
  tactual coding 173-5,
    182, 184, 186
  texture coding 176,
    193, 196
  verbal coding 173, 175,
    177, 178-82, 185
Braille writer 103
Braille writing 167-86
brain damage 5, 35, 44,
  see mental handicap
brain pathology 189

Callier-Azusa scale 116
caretaker 20-1, 62
  exchange with 111
  see mother, parents
caretaking behaviour 110
category systems 135-8
cerebral dysfunction 36
cerebral palsy 26-7
  see also mental handi-
  cap, multiple handicap
cluttering 31, see also
  language disorders
coding see phonological
  code, spatial coding,
  tactual coding, tex-
  ture coding, verbal
  coding
cognition 24, 133-41
  and language 16-17, 78,
    135, 140, 159-62
  social aspects 146

spatial 113
cognitive ability 14
cognitive complexity
  134
cognitive development
  78, 147
  blind children 114,
    131, 137-8, 142,
    144
  deaf children 137
  sighted children
    137-8
cognitive functioning
  142-61, 162
cognitive mechanisms 15
cognitive schemes 142
cognitive skills 50
cognitive theory
  language acquisition
    133-4
colour words 167, 185,
  189, see also visual
  terms
command
  obey inhibiting 11
communication 8, 12,
  107, 143
  gestural 129, see
  also gestures
  patterns of 109
  pre-linguistic 18
  pre-verbal 2, 114,
    143-4, 149, 159,
    160
  sensory systems 159
  situation 90
  verbal 18-41
communicative ability
  114
communicative acts 160
communicative aspects
  of language 145
communicative behaviour
  115, 120, 147
communicative compe-
  tence 108-13
communicative develop-
  ment 18, 108, 110,
  139
communicative function
  131, 143

communicative procedures
143, 158
communicative skills in-
terview 128-30
communicative systems 148,
165
communicative variables
139
compensatory behaviour 19
comprehension 46, 73, 80,
130, 185
concepts 21
deficient 69
development 7, 20, 63,
66, 72, 74
deviant 64
empty 185
formation 88
conceptual domains 75
conceptual input 142
conceptual level 188
conceptual problems 7
conceptual relations 143
conceptual structures 160
conceptual systems 78, 86
conceptual thought 187
conceptualization 81, 86-7,
161
congenitally blind
adult 164
children 26, 50, 59, 97,
116, 142, 147, 167-8,
175, 185
congenital visual defect
109
context
language and 154, 161
role of 63
speech 96, 104
conversational interchange
162, see dialogue
crawling
blind children 4-5, 7,
9-10, 116-19
see also locomotion,
motor skills

deaf children 57, 61, 86-7,
141, 164, 191-2
cognitive development
137

interaction 136
reading 170
sign language 141
deafness 26, 37, 134
deficit
language 86-7
language learning
74, 163
reading 190, 195
social 36
spatial 87, 191
deictics 95, 105, 111
see also gesture,
pointing
delay
acquisition of ref-
erence 131
acquisition of words
144-5
acquisition of word
combinations 145
cognitive develop-
ment 131, 138,
142, 152
communicative devel-
opment 108-11
development 1-2, 44,
116, 119, 146-7,
157-8, 163
and deviance 62, 163
language development
43, 59, 64,
111-12, 142, 195
object permanence
131
onset 64, 66
phonological acqui-
sition 60
speech 195
spontaneous use of
language 145
deprivation
maternal 3
sensory 3
deprived environment
196
development
blind children 13,
145, 157, 167
child 133-141
cognitive 78, 114,

131, 137-8, 142, 144
communicative 108-113
disorders 37
displaced reference
    96-7
ego 4
infant 144
intellectual 16
lexical 149
mental 26, 34, 43
phonology 22-3, 55-6, 60
physical 26, 34, 42
psychological 42
psycho-social 114
referential 89-107
semantic 90, 96, 104
syntax 21-2
theories of 146-7, 158
deviant communicative de-
    velopment 108-10
deviant language develop-
    ment 43, 56, 134
    see also delay, disor-
    ders
diagnosis 141
    handicap 29, 44
    language disorders 43
    visual impairment 117,
      119
diagnostic tests 140
dialogue
    blind adult 164
    blind children 142-61
    origins 110
    structuring by mother
      135
    sustaining devices 153
    verbal 7, 160
    vocal 19
    with words 6
disability
    communicative 163-4
    language 162-3
    linguistic 164
    phonetic 43
    specific linguistic
      165
discourse
    content 156
    context 94
    parent-child 161

skills 15
    see also interac-
    tion, verbal
    exchange
disorders
    see emotional dis-
    order, hearing dis-
    orders, language
    disorders, lexical
    disorders, morpho-
    syntactic disorders
    speech disorders
disturbed child 5
dyslexia 194-5

echolalia 21, 145, see
    also imitation,
    language disorders
educational programmes
    116-18, 127
    blind children 140,
      158
    see also interven-
    tion, speech
    therapy
educationally-subnor-
    mal 24, 30, 36
ego development 4, see
    also I, self
emotional disorder 26
emotional handicap 24
emotional relationship
    62
emotional tie 5, 10,
    see also affective
    tie
empiricism 74
English 16, 23, 50,
    55, 72, 82
experiment 69, 71, 85,
    168
experimental design
    78-9, see also
    methodology
expression
    blind children's
      facial 19, 114,
      121-3, 148, 153
    mothers' facial 120
expressive particles
    100

225

eye contact 58, 144, 148,
    see also gaze, regard
eye language 19, 114

first language acquisition
    13
form and function 160
formal structures 21.2,
    see also morphology,
    syntax
French 72
functions
    form and 160
    language 56, 89, 115,
        143-4, 158-60
    pre-verbal 160
fussing 115

gaze 62, 95, 150
    direction 94, 101-2
    reciprocal 162
    see also attention,
    eye contact, regard
German 16, 22-4, 42-3, 46,
    48, 50-1, 57
gestural communication
    128-9, 143
gestural complex 131
gesture 92, 95, 106, 145,
    149-50, 152
    blind children 121-9,
        131, 146, 153
    conventional 106-7,
        115, 120, 123, 129,
        131
    infant 125-7
    non-conventional 128-9
    referential 111, 128
    sighted children 115,
        160
glaucoma 147
grapheme 61
    -phoneme correspondence
        rules 170
    -phoneme translation
        194
greeting terms 100

hand language 114
handicap
    blindness as 72, 88

concomitant 5, 112,
    117, see multiply-
    handicapped
degree 109, see also
    visual faculty
language 62, 66, see
    also delay, lan-
    guage disorders
onset 18, see also
    diagnosis
physical 36
sensory 116
visual 163
haptic activity 69
haptic meanings 87
haptic modality 81
haptic verbs 74, 80
hearing 50, 81
    disorders 36
    impairment 44
    see also deaf
Hungarian 23
hypotonia 116

I
    concept 2
    /you distinction 12,
        56
    see also ego develop-
    ment, self/other dif-
    ferentiation
illusions 47-8, 159
imagery 69
images 9
imaginative thought 12
imitation 42, 49
    adults 95, 124
    blind children 20-2,
        118-19, 121,
        128-9, 145, 149
    elicited 50-1
    sighted children 115
impaired language
    learner 13-17
impairment
    visual 26, 107, 110,
        113, 117, 119
    see also blindness,
    handicap
infant behaviours 115,
    119-20, 125, 135

infant vocalization 124-7
innate ability 59
innate mechanism 133
institutionalized babies
    4
intellectual development
    16
intelligence 6, 14
    quotient 175-7, 179,
        194
    representational 1-2
    sensori-motor 143, 145
interaction 111, 114-132,
    143
    blind children 106,
        114-133, 136, 150-1,
        153
    caretaker-child 110
    coding system 119-121
    deaf children 136
    initiation 150-1
    and language 136
    mother-child 119,
        124-8, 133-41, 149,
        154
    parent-child 112, 148,
        159
    patterns 114-32
    reciprocal 146
    sequences 153
    topic of 130
interactive theory 133-4
intervention 132, 140-1,
    145, 158, 164
    procedures 113, 190-6
    programmes 187-196
interview 128, see also
    methodology
intonation 118, 149, 156,
    167

knowledge
    conceptual 189-90
    listener's 97
    real world 188
    semantic 189-90
    shared 93, 102
    spatial 80-1

language
    of the blind 78, 189

blind children 11, 62
    and cognition 16-17,
        78, 135, 140,
        159-62
    deficient 87
    emergence 144, 149
    and thought 160
language abnormalities
    24-40
    classification 27-34
    frequency of 27-34
    incidence 24-27
    see also language
    disorders
language acquisition 16,
    49, 156
    blind children 89-90
    conditions for 134
    deficient 163
    normal 158, 164
    sighted children
        89-90, 142-3, 146
    theories 133-4
language development 10,
    58
    blind children 12, 34,
        56, 59, 131, 162
    delay 43, 59, 64,
        111-12, 142, 195
    deviant 43, 56, 134
    level 152
    measure 89
    pathological 42, 44
    retardation 37, 56
language deviations 62
    see also deviant lan-
    guage development
language disorders
    24-38, 42-3, 56
    multiple 31
    partially-sighted
        children 24-38
    sighted children 28,
        31-2
    totally blind children
        24-38
    see also language ab-
    normalities, deficit,
    delay, deviance
language learning 63, 75
    deficit 74

situation 14
language problems 42,
145, 166, see language
abnormalities, lan-
guage disorders
language skills 118, 128
language system 81
lateralization see Braille,
hand advantage
Leber's amaurosis 97
Leber's tapetoretinal de-
generation 50
letter
discrimination 176
naming 176
see Braille, Braille
reading, Braille writing
lexical deficiency 87
lexical development 149
lexical distinction 75
lexical field 44
lexical level 188
lexical-semantic disorders
31, 35, 37, 39
lexical substitutions 87
lexicon 42-3, 77, 170, 182
linguistic ability 114
linguistic deficit 86
linguistic development 26,
42-3, 165, see language
development
linguistic level 66, 76
linguistic vocalization 123
lip
movements 23, 57, 59
positions 49
see articulation
lip-reading 46, 51, 57-61
listener's ability to
interpret 106
listening 127, 150
location markers 154
locative actions 66
locative states 66
locomotion 1-2
locomotor abilities 131, see
also crawling, motor de-
velopment, walking
longitudinal study
blind children 97, 115,
139, 142, 151, 153

see also methodolo-
gy

manual activity
blind children 116,
121, 123
see also hand lan-
guage
maturation, physio-
logical 8
maternal behaviour
119, 125, see
mother, parents
maternal vocalization
125-7
meaning
acquisition 20,
77-88
deviation 63
errors 96, 105
relations 144
in syntactic utter-
ances 66
theories 78
word 63, 72-3, 75,
77, 80, 84, 107,
160-1, 170, 182,
188
see also semantics
meaningless language
62-76, 85, 87, 170,
see also semantic-
ally empty words,
verbalism
memory 81, 88, 93, 184
conceptual 188
reading 176
semantic 188
tactual impressions
182, 186
verbal 178
mental deficiency 37
mental development 26,
34, 43
mental handicap 26,
34, 36, 164
mental retardation 44
mentalistic theory
133-4
methodology 13-14, 80,
109, 135, 138-9,

see also experiment, longitudinal study, observation, statistical analysis
midline, hands at 4, 9, 116
MLU 64, 76, 112
mobility 5
  spatial 113
  see also locomotion, motor development
modality 70, 83, 87, 168
  auditory 49, 57
  haptic 81
  optic 81
  sense 86
  touch 80, 85
  visual 49, 57, 78
morphology 21, 42, 44
morpho-syntactic disorders 33-43
mother
  adaptability 139-40
  behaviours 135
  -child interaction 119, 124-8, 133-41, 149, 154
  preference for 4
  speech 153
  see also maternal behaviour, parents
motivation
  effectance 108-13
motor changes 9
motor development 7, 20, 114
motor skills 50, 118
multiply-handicapped children 20-37 passim
muscular dystrophy 36

naming 151-4, 157
nasality 31
  see also rhinolalia
negation 16, 66
negatives 85
neonate
  signalling abilities 115
  receptive abilities 115

neurological damage 145, 147, see also multiply-handicapped children
non-linguistic noise 99
non-linguistic sound 121
non-spatial coding 172, 182, see also Braille reading, tactual code
non-verbal behaviour 111
non-verbal communications 2
non-verbal context 96
non-verbal devices 93, 100, 105, 107
non-verbal dialogue 5
non-verbal infant behaviour 120
non-verbal mechanisms 130
non-verbal strategies 92, 96, 99, 102
non-visual systems 159
non-vocal sound 121-2, 135
nouns, acquisition 64
object permanence 2, 62, 131, 146, 150, 152
observation 69, 136-40 passim, see also methodology
one-word stage 64, 143-51
onset
  delay 64, 66
  language 64
  visual impairment 26
  see also language emergence
optic aphasia 189
optic atrophy 147
optic hypoplasia 117
optic modality 81
optic nerve, deformity 64
over-extensions 149, see also semantic development

parental treatment 75

parental vocalization 132, see also vocalization
parents
    blind children 106, 111, 147-51
    see also caretaker, mother
partially-sighted children
    communicative competence 108, 112-13
    language disorders 24-38 *passim*
    sample 44
    teaching 40
perception 42, 47, 49, 58, 88
    definition 86
    experiments 46
    modes 21, 72
    speech sounds 23, 46
    tactile-haptic 71-2, 75
    verbs 69, 72-3, 78, 81, 83
    see also modality
perceptual processing 15
perceptual system 86
Perkins key-board 176, 181
    see also Braille
personal-social words acquisition 64
phonemic route 193-4, see reading
phonetic disability 43
phonetics 42
phonology 42, 59-60
    development 22-3, 55-6, 60, 110
    deviant 15
    sighted children 59
phonological abnormalities 23, 31
phonological acquisition 15, 49, 57-61
phonological code 61, 170
phonological disorders 33-43 *passim*, 59-61, see also language disorders
phonological output 60
phonological route 194 see reading

phonological rules 56
phonological substitutions 46-56, 59
phonological system 61, 182
physical development 26, 34, 42
physical environment 110
physical handicap 36, see also handicap
play
    blind children 6, 128-9
    social 152
pointing 95, 102, 111, 115, 130, 145, 150, see also attention, gesture
possession relation 155, 157
pragmatic information 49
pragmatic problems 40
pragmatics 115, 128
precursors
    articulatory movements 23
    formal language 115
    language development 1-12, 13-17
    reference 107
    verbal exchange 128
predicate-argument structure 63-4
predictor of language development 130
prehension 2
pre-linguistic communication 18
pre-linguistic period 95
pre-linguistic roots of language 89
prematurity 3, 64
pre-referential development 94
pre-verbal ability 114-5
pre-verbal behaviour 115, 127

230

pre-verbal communication 2, 114, 143-4, 149, 158, 160
pre-verbal functions 160
pre-verbal infant 100, 189
pre-verbal period 146, 148, 152-3, 159
pre-verbal procedures 145
pre-verbal stage 22
pre-verbal vocalizations 149
production 42, 59, 73, 130
propositional content of utterances 143, 145
proprioception 61
prosodic marking 148, see also intonation
psychological development 42
psycho-social development 114

questions 85, 100
    acquisition of 154
    adults' 111-12
    for assessing attention 101, 105
    referring 105

reach
    on sight 4
    on sound 4, 119
    see also auditory localization skills
reading
    blind children 167-86
    deficit 190, 195
    difficulties in aphasia 193
    hemispheres involved 174
    retardation 195
    tactual 180-1
    visual 172, 180-1, 184, 186
    visual, model of 170
    see also Braille, Braille reading,
    dyslexia
reference 152, 154
    acquisition 15, 21, 131
    ambiguity 164
    displaced 93, 96-7
    establishment 90, 130-1
    external 131
    frame 144
    mutual 62
    to objects 155, 163
    see also referential development
referential act 90-6, 163
referential development 89-107
    sighted children 94-7
referential function 89-90, 94, 97
referential problems 105
referring expressions 89-96, 104-5
    definite conditions on 104
regard
    direction of 110-11
    visual 115, 120
    see also attention, eye contact, gaze
representation
    abstract 71
    concrete objects 20
    emergence 145, 150, 152, 158
    iconic 80
    self 146
    see also object permanence
representational capacity 74
representational intelligence 1-2
requests 146, 152, 155, 157, 159
retardation
    Braille reading 170, 175, 178-80
    cognitive development 137
    development 5, 36

general reading 195
language development
    26, 37, 56
    see also delay,
    deviance
retrolental fibroplasia
    3, 64, 97
Russian 23
sample 43-4, 108-9, 112
    see also methodology
self
    concept of 131
    /other differentia-
        tion 8, 128, 131,
        156
    representation 146
    see also I
semantic aspects of lan-
    guage 145
semantic content 85
semantic components 77,
    81
semantic development 90,
    96, 104, see also
    meaning acquisition
semantic differential 69
semantic distinctions 83
semantic encoding 187,
    189
semantic field 44
semantic incongruity 167
semantic information 49
semantic knowledge 188
semantic level 188
semantic primes 78
semantic problem 40
semantic relations 66,
    151, 160
semantic route in read-
    ing 194
semantic rules 189
semantic-syntactic rela-
    tions 76
semantic system 80, 172,
    186
semantic theories 187-96
semantically empty words
    187, see also meaning-
    less language, verbal-
    ism
semantics 42-3, 89, 142,

144
sense
    modality 86
    percept 81
sensorially-deprived
    children 86
sensorially-handicapped
    87
sensorium 75
sensory apparatus 74
sensory communication
    systems 159
sensory experience 63,
    66, 72, 159
sensory handicap 116
sensory input 69, 81, 86
sensory language 78
sensory system 87
separation anxiety 11
shape coding, reading
    174, see also Braille
sighted children
    development of refer-
        ence 94-7
    expressed meanings
        64-9
    gesture 115, 160
    imitation 21, 115
    language acquisition
        89-90, 142-3, 146
    language disorders
        28, 31-2
    phonology 59
    referential develop-
        ment 94-7
sighted children studied
    Amahl 50, 52-55
    Elaine 148, 155-6
    Joanna 50-54
    Patty 3-4, 10
sighted terms, use of
    159, see vision
    verbs, visual verbs,
    visual words
sign systems 135-6, see
    interaction
silence 127
smile 4-5, 10
    infant 124-7, 139
    language 18, 114
    see also expression

social aspects of cog-
    nition 146
social class 35, 37
social conditions 26
social deficit 36
social environment 110
social factors 26, 195
social interaction 145,
    148, 161
social milieu 23, 26
social play 152
social situation 92
social skills 118
sonar for the blind 87
space
    exploration 122
    navigation 62
    orientation 73, 75
spatial coding 170,
    175-6, 178-81, 186,
    190-3, 196, see
    also Braille reading
spatial cognition 113
spatial deficit 87, 191
spatial knowledge 80-1
spatial mobility 113
spatial relationships
    20
spatial system 87
spatial tasks 178
speaker-listener dyad
    92, 194
speech
    almost no 33-4, 38
    spontaneous 59
    see also disorders
speech abnormalities 23
speech act theory 143,
    see also functions
    of language,
    pragmatics
speech disorders 43
speech perception 57,
    59-61
    models 46, 49
    Motor theory 61
speech problems 114
    see speech disorders
speech sounds 21, 57,
    59
    acoustic properties

49
    acquisition 46-56
    perception 23, 46
speech therapy 22, 27,
    31, 39-40, 42-5, see
    also educational pro-
    grammes, intervention
spontaneous production
    130
spontaneous speech 59
spontaneous use of lan-
    guage 145
spontaneous utterances
    50-1, 53-4
spontaneous vocalizations
    114
stammering 33, 38, see
    also language disor-
    ders, speech disorders
statistical analysis
    136-40
statistical evidence 195
    see also methodology
stranger reaction 4
structure 56, 73
    syntactic 143
    see also form, syntax
stuttering 31
subjects
    small numbers 79
    see sample
Switzerland 28
syntactic abilities 114
syntactic behaviour 86
syntactic contexts 80-1
syntactic function 85
syntactic learning 63
syntactic structure 143
syntactic utterances 76
syntax 42, 44, 73
    acquisition 133
    development 21

tactile behaviour 121
tactile exploration 119,
    see touch
tactile/haptic perception
    71-2, 75
tactual coding 173-5,
    182, 184, 186, see
    also Braille reading

tactual reading 180-1,
    see also Braille
    reading
temporal coding 191
tense markers 97
texture coding 176, 193,
    196, see also Braille
    reading
totally blind 3, 25, 37,
    44, 108, 116, 147,
    150-1, 167-8, 185
    language disorders in
        28-38 passim
    see also partially-
    sighted, visual
    faculty
touch
    active 167-86
    maternal 122, 125-7
    modality 80, 85
touching
    directing attention
        95, 99, 102
    mothers' 119, 123,
        139, 148
    see also touch
turn-taking 112, 115,
    130, 149
two-word utterances 12,
    50, see also syntax,
    word combination

unresponsiveness, blind
    children 10

verbal coding 173, 175
    177
    in reading 178-82,
        185
    see also Braille
    reading
verbal communication
    143, 149
    abnormalities 18-41
verbal devices in ref-
    erential develop-
    ment 95-6, 100,
    105-7
verbal dialogue 7
verbal infant behaviour
    120

verbal interaction 133
verbal strategies 103
    mediating other skills
        167, 170, 172, 176,
        181, 185-6, 190
verbal system 184
verbal tests 178
verbalism 21, 63, 66, 69,
    85-6, 104, 161, 167,
    185, 187, see also
    meaningless language
viseme 46, see visually-
    distinctive sound
vision
    lack 63, 157
    limited 147
    role 1-2, 40, 59, 90,
        95, 107, 144,
        157-62
    verbs 72, 85
    see also blind chil-
    dren, partially-sight-
    ed children, sighted
    terms, visual verbs
visual category 60
visual cues 84, 101
visual exchanges 124
visual experience 63, 74
    see also sensory ex-
    perience
visual faculty 26, 30, 33
    see also blind chil-
    dren, blindness,
    handicap, partially-
    sighted children,
    visual impairment
visual group of sounds
    47-56, see also
    viseme, visually-dis-
    tinctive sounds
visual handicap 163
visual impairment 26,
    107, 110, 113, 117,
    119, see also blind
    children, blindness,
    diagnosis, onset, par-
    tially-sighted chil-
    dren, visually-
    impaired
visual information 46-9,
    see also articulatory

movements
visual language 86, see
    visual terms
visual modality 49, 57,
    78
visual system 87
visual terminology 64,
    74-5, see also sighted
    terms, visual terms,
    visual words
visual terms 69, 78, 168,
    187
visual verbs 69, see
    vision verbs
visual words 73, 104, see
    also visual terms
visually-distinctive
    sounds 46, 48, 59, see
    also viseme, visual
    group
visually-handicapped 18
visually-impaired children
    abnormalities in com-
        munication 18-40
    see also blind chil-
    dren, partially-sighted
    children
visually-perceived attrib-
    ute 104
vocabulary 63-4, 76, 96,
    114, 128, 150, see also
    lexicon, semantics
vocal dialogue 19, see
    dialogue
vocal exchange 124, 127
vocal patterns 132
vocal sounds 3
vocalization 2, 5, 11,
    94-5, 118-19, 122, 131,
    148
    child's reaction to 135
    imitation of 129
    infant 124-7
    linguistic 123
    maternal 125-7
    mothers' 118-19, 122,
        124, 135
    mothers' reaction to
        135
    non-linguistic 125
    parental 132

rate 122, 128
responses to 132
spontaneous 114
vocative 100, 105

walking, blind children
    4, 7, 9, 11-12, 118,
    131, see also crawl-
    ing, locomotion,
    locomotor abilities,
    motor development
Wasco 72
word association 69
word combinations 20,
    143-4, 148, 150, see
    also syntax, two-word
    utterances
words
    first 11, 149
    see also one-word
    stage
writing 167-86, see
    Braille, Braille key-
    board, Braille writer